American College of
Emergency Physicians®

Pocket
First Aid

D0835163

DK

LONDON, NEW YORK, MUNICH,
MELBOURNE, DELHI

SENIOR EDITOR Janet Mohun
US SENIOR EDITOR Jill Hamilton
ART EDITOR Sara Freeman
DTP DESIGNER Julian Dams
SENIOR MANAGING EDITOR Jemima Dunne
MANAGING ART EDITOR Louise Dick
PRODUCTION CONTROLLER Louise Daly
PRODUCTION MANAGER Sarah Coltman

Produced for DK Publishing by
COOLING BROWN
9–11 High St, Hampton, Middlesex TW12 2SA

First published in the United States in 2003 by
DK Publishing, Inc.
375 Hudson Street,
New York, New York 10014

00 01 02 03 04 05 10 9 8 7 6 5 4 3 2 1

Illustration copyright © 2003 by
Dorling Kindersley Limited

Text copyright © 2003 by St. John Ambulance;
St. Andrew's Ambulance Association; The British
Red Cross Society

Pocket first aid / American College of Emergency
Physicians ; medical editor, Jon R. Krohmer MD
p. cm.   Includes index.
ISBN 0-7894-9265-2 (alk. paper)
1. First aid in illness and injury--Handbooks,
manuals, etc. I. Krohmer, Jon R. II.
American College of Emergency Physicians.
RC86.8.P644 2003
616.02'52--dc21   2002073597

Reproduced in Singapore by Colourscan

Printed and bound by South China
Printing Co. Ltd., China

See our complete catalog at
www.dk.com

CONTENTS

5 BONE, JOINT, AND MUSCLE INJURIES   69

6 DISORDERS OF CONSCIOUSNESS   87

7 ENVIRONMENTAL INJURIES   97

8 FOREIGN OBJECTS   111

9 POISONING, BITES, AND STINGS   117

INTRODUCTION

Pocket First Aid covers essential first-aid techniques in detail in a compact format that is readily accessible at a medical emergency. The book gives clear and comprehensive step-by-step advice on first-aid treatments, from life-saving resuscitation procedures to dressing wounds.

The information in this book is based on guidelines for first-aid treatments and resuscitation methods that were agreed upon in 2000 by the American Heart Association, the Heart and Stroke Foundation of Canada, the European Resuscitation Council, and other national and international

organizations. The material in this manual provides guidance on initial care and treatment; however, it should not be regarded as a substitute for medical advice.

The American College of Emergency Physicians does not accept responsibility for any claims arising from the use of this manual, even if the guidelines given here have been followed.

First aiders are advised to obtain training from a qualified instructor and to keep up to date with developments by periodic recertification. In addition, first aiders should always recognize the limits of their own competence.

HOW TO USE THIS BOOK

Color bars help you find relevant sections quickly

Introductory text describes likely causes and effects of condition

"Your aims" box summarizes purposes of treatment

Annotated photographs show details of particular techniques

Steps explain each stage of first-aid action

SWALLOWED POISONS

Chemicals that are swallowed may harm the digestive tract, or cause more widespread damage if they enter the bloodstream. Hazardous chemicals include common household substances such as bleach, dishwasher detergent, and paint thinner.

Drugs, whether prescribed or bought over the counter, are also potentially harmful if they are taken in overdose. The effects of poisoning depend on the substance that has been swallowed.

YOUR AIMS
- To maintain the airway, breathing, and circulation.
- To remove any contaminated clothing.
- To identify the poison.
- To arrange urgent removal to the hospital

1 If the victim is conscious, ask her what she has swallowed, and try to reassure her.

Look for clues such as empty containers.

2 CALL THE POISON CONTROL CENTER (800) 222-1222
Give as much information as possible about the swallowed poison, to help the doctors to give appropriate treatment once the victim reaches the hospital.

118

RECOGNITION
Depends on the poison, but there may be:
- Vomiting, sometimes bloodstained.
- Impaired consciousness.
- Pain or burning sensation.
- Empty containers in the vicinity.
- History of ingestion/exposure

See also CHEMICAL BURN p.103 • DRUG POISONING p.119 • LIFE-SAVING PROCEDURES pp.19–48

SPECIAL CASE
BURNED LIPS
If the victim's lips are burned by corrosive substances, give her cold milk or water to rinse her mouth while waiting for medical help.

WARNING
- Never attempt to induce vomiting.
- If the victim becomes unconscious, open the airway and check breathing; be prepared to give rescue breaths and chest compressions if necessary (see LIFE-SAVING PROCEDURES, pp.19–48).
- If she is breathing, place her in the recovery position (pp.30–31).

- Use a face shield or pocket mask (p.24) for rescue breathing if there are any chemicals on the victim's mouth.

List of recognition features provides quick-reference guide to help you identify condition

Cross-references direct you to articles on related conditions or further treatment

"Special case" box highlights instances in which alternative action may be needed

"Warning" box advises on dealing with dangers and avoiding further risks to victim or yourself

4

ACTION AT AN EMERGENCY

By working according to a clear plan, you will be able to prioritize the demands that may be made on you in any emergency situation. Avoid placing yourself in danger, be aware of hazards such as oil or gas, and do not attempt to do too much by yourself.

FIRST-AID PRIORITIES

● *Assess the situation.* Quickly and calmly observe what has happened, and look for dangers to yourself, the victim, and any bystanders. Consider whether anyone's life is in immediate danger; if there are bystanders who could help; and whether you need specialized assistance.

● *Make the area safe.* Conditions that gave rise to the incident may present a danger. Put your own safety first. Simple measures, such as turning off a switch, can often make the area safe.
● *Give emergency aid.* Assess all victims to determine treatment priorities, and treat those with life-threatening conditions first. Establish whether the victim is conscious, check whether his airway is open and whether he is breathing, and look for signs of circulation.
● *Get help from others.* Check that any necessary medical aid or other expert help has been called and is on its way.

TELEPHONING FOR HELP

You can summon help by telephone from a number of sources.
● **Emergency services** (dial 9·1·1 or call your local EMS): police, fire, and emergency medical services.
● **Utilities:** gas, electricity, or water.
● **Health services:** doctor or dentist.
● **Poison Control Center** (dial 800-222-1222): suspected poison. Emergency calls are free and can be made on any telephone, including car phones and cellular phones.

WHAT TO TELL EMERGENCY SERVICES

State your name, that you are a first aider, and give the following details:
● Your telephone number.
● The location of the incident; give a road name or number, if possible, and any junctions or other landmarks.
● The type of incident; for example, "Traffic collision, two cars, road blocked, three people trapped."
● The number, sex, and approximate ages of the victims, and what you know about their condition.
● Details of any hazardous substances, such as gas, or relevant weather conditions, such as fog or ice.

Calling the emergency services
Try to stay calm so that you can give all the information the emergency services need. Let the dispatcher hang up first.

LOOKING AFTER YOURSELF

When giving first aid, particularly if you are treating open wounds, it is important to prevent "cross infection" (transmitting germs to a victim or contracting an infection yourself).

Often, simple measures, such as washing your hands and wearing disposable gloves, provide sufficient protection. There is a risk of infection with blood-borne viruses such as hepatitis B or C and Human Immunodeficiency Virus (HIV), but these viruses can only be transmitted by blood-to-blood contact – if an infected person's blood makes contact with yours through, for example, a cut or scrape.

Protection from hepatitis B
All first aiders should be protected against hepatitis B by immunization. The vaccine is given as a series of three injections in the upper arm.

IMMUNIZATION
It is recommended that all first aiders are immunized against hepatitis B Currently, there is no vaccine against hepatitis C or HIV. If you think you have been exposed to any infection after giving first aid, seek medical aid immediately.

GUIDELINES FOR PREVENTING CROSS INFECTION

Following good practice guidelines will help prevent infection.
● If possible, wash your hands in soap and water before treating a victim.
● Carry protective disposable gloves with you and use them when you are giving treatment. If gloves are not available, ask the victim to dress his own wound, or enclose your hands in clean plastic bags.
● Cover cuts and scrapes on your hands with waterproof dressings.
● Wear a plastic apron and plastic glasses when dealing with quantities of body fluids.
● Avoid touching a wound or any part of a dressing that will come into contact with a wound.

● Try not to breathe, cough, or sneeze over a wound while treating a victim.
● Be extremely careful not to prick yourself with any needle found on or near a victim, or cut yourself on glass.
● If a face shield or pocket mask is available, use it when you are giving rescue breaths (p.24).
● Dispose of waste safely. Place soiled items in a plastic bag, ideally a special yellow biohazard bag, which should then be sealed and incinerated.

> **❶ WARNING**
> If you accidentally prick or cut your skin or splash your eyes, wash the area thoroughly and seek medical help immediately.

1

T HIS CHAPTER outlines the core procedures that are central to the practice of first aid. Techniques for assessing a victim are outlined first, followed by a guide to materials that make up a useful first-aid kit, and how to use them. Finally, the application of various kinds of dressings and bandages is shown and explained. This is a critical part of effective first aid because wounds usually require a dressing, and most injuries benefit from the support of bandages.

CONTENTS

TECHNIQUES AND EQUIPMENT

FIRST-AID PRIORITIES

- Assess the victim's condition.
- Comfort and reassure the victim.
- Remove clothing if necessary.
- Use a first-aid technique relevant to the injury.
- Use dressings and bandages as needed.
- Monitor and record level of response, pulse, and breathing.
- Obtain medical aid if necessary. Dial 9·1·1 or call your local EMS at once if you suspect a serious illness or injury.

MONITORING VITAL SIGNS

When you are treating a victim, you may need to assess and monitor his level of response, pulse, and breathing. You may also need to monitor his temperature. These vital signs may help you identify specific problems and indicate changes in a victim's condition. Monitoring should be repeated regularly and your findings recorded on an observation chart (p.128), which should be handed to the medical team taking over.

CHECKING LEVEL OF RESPONSE

You will need to monitor a victim's level of response in order to assess consciousness. Any injury or illness that affects the brain may affect consciousness, and deterioration in response is potentially serious.

Assess the victim's level of response using the AVPU code:
A – Is the victim *Alert*? Does the victim open his eyes and respond to questions?

V – Does the victim respond to *Voice*? Does he answer simple questions and obey commands?
P – Does the victim respond to *Pain*? Does he open his eyes or move if he is pinched?
U – Is the victim *Unresponsive* to any stimulus?

Using this code, you can check whether there is any change in the victim's condition.

CHECKING PULSE

The normal pulse rate in adults is 60–80 beats per minute. The rate is faster in children and may be slower in very fit adults. An abnormally fast or slow pulse may be a sign of certain illnesses. The pulse may be measured at the neck (carotid pulse) or the wrist (radial pulse). In babies, the pulse in the upper arm (brachial pulse) may be easier to find.

When checking a pulse, use your fingers rather than your thumb (which has its own pulse), and press lightly until you can feel the pulse. Record the following points:
• Rate (the number of beats per minute).
• Strength (strong or weak).
• Rhythm (regular or irregular).

Brachial pulse
Place two fingers on the inner side of the infant's upper arm.

Use pads of your fingers

Radial pulse
Place three fingers at the base of the thumb just below the creases of the wrist.

Carotid pulse
Place two fingers on the side of the neck, in the hollow between the windpipe and the large neck muscle.

CHECKING BREATHING

When assessing a victim's breathing, check the rate of breathing, listen for breathing difficulties or noises, and watch the victim's chest movements. The normal breathing rate in adults is 12–16 breaths per minute; in babies and young children, it is 20–30 breaths per minute. For a baby or young child, place your hand on the chest and feel for breathing. Record the following:

- Rate (number of breaths per minute).
- Depth (deep or shallow breaths).
- Ease (whether breaths are easy, difficult, or painful).
- Noise (whether breathing is quiet or noisy, and types of noise).

Feel rise and fall of child's chest as he breathes

Use a watch to time breaths per minute

Assessing breathing rate
Watch the chest move and count the number of breaths per minute. For a baby or young child, it may be easier if you place your hand on the chest.

CHECKING TEMPERATURE

To assess body temperature, feel the exposed skin and obtain an accurate reading using a thermometer. Normal body temperature is 98.6°F (37°C). A high temperature (fever) is usually caused by infection. A low body temperature (hypothermia) may result from exposure to cold and/or wet conditions. There are several types of thermometer, including traditional glass mercury and digital models; make sure that you know how to use them.

Digital thermometer
This can be used to measure temperature under the tongue or under the armpit. Leave it in place until it makes a beeping sound (about 30 seconds), then read the temperature from the display.

Forehead thermometer
The heat-sensitive strip is useful for a young child, but it is not as accurate as the digital thermometer. Hold the strip against the child's forehead for about 30 seconds. The color indicates the temperature.

Mercury thermometer
Before using this thermometer check that the mercury level is below 98.6°F (37°C). Leave the thermometer in position (under the tongue or in the armpit) for 2–3 minutes before reading.

Ear sensor
Place the tip of this thermometer inside the ear; it will give a reading within 1 second. The sensor is easy to use and is very useful for a vomiting child; however, it is not as accurate as a digital one.

FIRST-AID MATERIALS

All workplaces, recreational centers, homes, and cars should have first-aid kits. The kits for workplaces or recreational centers must conform to legal requirements; they should also be clearly marked and easily accessible. For a home or a car, you can either buy a kit or assemble first-aid items yourself and keep them in a clean, waterproof container. First-aid kits must be kept in a dry place, and checked and replenished regularly.

The items on these pages (see also p.12) form the basis of a home first-aid kit. You may wish to add items such as aspirin and acetaminophen.

DRESSINGS

Fabric adhesive bandages

Waterproof adhesive bandages

Clear adhesive bandages

Heel and finger adhesive bandages

Adhesive bandages or dressings
These items are applied to small cuts and scrapes and are made of fabric or waterproof plastic. Waterproof types are best for hand wounds, and hypoallergenic types for anyone who is allergic to the adhesive in normal wear. People who work with food are required to use blue adhesive bandages.

Eye pad

Eye pad with headband

Sterile eye pads
Eye pads are dressings that are used to protect injured eyes. Some eye pads have headbands attached so that they can be secured to a victim's head.

Medium dressing

Large dressing

Extra-large dressing

Sterile dressings
These consist of a dressing pad attached to a roller bandage, and are sealed in a protective wrapping. They are easy to apply, and thus are ideal in an emergency. Various sizes are available.

BANDAGES

Self-adhesive
roller bandage

Crêpe roller
bandage

Open-weave roller
bandage

Roller bandages
These items are used to give support to injured joints, restrict movement, secure dressings in place and maintain pressure on them, and limit swelling.

Elasticized roller
bandage

Conforming roller
bandage

Crêpe conforming
roller bandage

Folded cloth
triangular bandage

Folded paper
triangular bandage

Triangular bandages
Made of cloth or strong paper, these items can be used as bandages and slings. If they are sterile and individually wrapped, they may also be used as dressings for large wounds and burns.

BASIC MATERIALS FOR A HOME FIRST-AID KIT

- Easily identifiable watertight box.
- 20 adhesive bandages or dressings in assorted sizes.
- Two crêpe roller bandages.
- Six medium sterile dressings.
- Two large sterile dressings.
- Two extra-large sterile dressings.
- Two sterile eye pads.
- Six triangular bandages.
- Six safety pins.
- Disposable gloves.

Useful additions:
- Scissors.
- Tweezers.
- Cotton.
- Nonalcoholic cleansing wipes.
- Adhesive tape.
- Plastic face shield or pocket face mask.
- Notepad, pencil, and tags.
- Blanket, survival bag, flashlight, and whistle.

FIRST-AID MATERIALS (continued)

ADDITIONAL ITEMS FOR A HOME FIRST-AID KIT

Gauze pads
Use these as dressings, padding, or as swabs to clean around wounds.

Cleansing wipes
Alcohol-free wipes can be used to clean skin around wounds, or to clean your hands if water and soap are not available.

Disposable gloves
Wear gloves, if available, especially when dressing wounds or handling body fluids or other waste materials.

Face protection
When giving rescue breaths, use a plastic face shield (left) or a pocket mask (right) to protect you and the victim from infections.

Bandage clip

Safety pins

Pins and clips
These items can be used to secure the ends of bandages.

COLD COMPRESSES

Cooling an injury such as a bruise or sprain can reduce swelling and pain, although it will not relieve the injury itself. There are two types of compress: cold pads, which are materials dampened with cold water; and ice packs, which are cold items (such as ice cubes or packs of frozen peas or other vegetables) wrapped in a dry cloth.

COLD PAD

1 Soak a washcloth or towel in very cold water. Wring it out lightly, fold it into a pad, and place it firmly on the injury.

2 Resoak the pad in cold water every 3–5 minutes to keep it cold. Apply it to the injury for at least 10 minutes.

ICE PACK

1 Partly fill a plastic bag with small ice cubes or crushed ice, or use a pack of frozen vegetables. Wrap the bag in a dry cloth.

2 Hold the pack firmly on the area for 10 minutes, replacing the pack as needed.

Cover injury and surrounding area with pack

> **! CAUTION**
>
> To prevent cold injuries, always wrap an ice pack in a cloth, and do not use it for more than 10 minutes at one application.

STERILE DRESSINGS

This type of dressing consists of a dressing pad attached to a roller bandage. The pad is a piece of gauze backed by a layer of cotton.

Sterile dressings are sold individually in various sizes and they are sealed in protective wrappings to prevent contamination. Once the seal on this type of dressing has been broken, the dressing is no longer sterile.

❶ CAUTION

- If the dressing slips out of place, remove it and apply a new dressing.
- If bleeding appears through the dressing, apply another on top of the original one. If blood seeps through the second dressing as well, take off both dressings and apply a fresh one.
- Take care not to restrict the circulation beyond the dressing.

1 Break the seal and remove the wrapping. Unwind the bandage, taking care not to drop the roll or touch the pad.

2 Unfold the dressing pad, holding the bandage on each side of it. Lay the pad directly on the wound.

Use a pad that is larger than wound

3 Wind the short end (tail) of the bandage once around the limb and the dressing to secure the pad.

Head of bandage

Tail of bandage

4 Wind the other end (head) of the bandage around the limb to cover the whole pad. Leave the tail of the bandage hanging free.

Head of bandage

Tail of bandage

5 To secure the bandage, tie the ends in a square knot (p.16). Tie the knot directly over the pad to exert firm pressure on the wound.

Ensure that bandage covers dressing pad completely

Tie square knot over dressing pad

6 Once you have secured the bandage, check the circulation in the limb beyond it (p.14). Loosen the bandage if it is too tight.

PRINCIPLES OF BANDAGING

There are a number of different first-aid uses for bandages: they can be used to secure dressings, control bleeding, support and immobilize limbs, and reduce swelling in an injured part. If you do not have a bandage, you can improvise one from an everyday item; for example, you can fold a square of lightweight fabric, such as a scarf, diagonally to make a triangular bandage (p.16).

▶ See also ROLLER BANDAGES opposite
● TRIANGULAR BANDAGES p.16

RULES FOR APPLYING A BANDAGE

● Make the victim comfortable, in a suitable sitting or lying position, and explain what you are going to do.
● Keep the injured part supported while you are working on it. Ask the victim or a helper to do this.
● Work at the front of the victim, and from the injured side if possible.
● If the victim is lying down, pass the bandages under hollows at the ankles, knees, waist, and neck, then slide the bandages back and forth under the body into position.
● Tie bandages with square knots (p.16).
● Leave the fingers or toes on a bandaged limb exposed, if possible.
● Regularly check the circulation in the area beyond the bandage (below). If necessary, unroll the bandage until the blood supply returns, and reapply it more loosely.

CHECKING CIRCULATION AFTER BANDAGING

When bandaging a limb or using a sling, check the circulation in the hand or foot immediately after you have finished bandaging, and every 10 minutes thereafter. These checks are essential because limbs swell after an injury, and a bandage can rapidly become too tight and interfere with blood circulation to the area beyond it. Symptoms of impaired circulation change as first the veins and then the arteries become constricted.

RECOGNITION
If circulation is impaired there may be:
● A swollen and congested limb.
● Blue skin with prominent veins.
● A feeling that the skin is painfully distended.
Later there may be:
● Pale, waxy skin.
● Cold numbness.
● Tingling, followed by deep pain.
● Inability to move affected fingers or toes.

1 Briefly press one of the nails, or the skin, until it turns pale, then release the pressure. If the color does not return, or returns slowly, the bandage may be too tight.

2 Loosen a tight bandage by unrolling just enough turns for warmth and color to return to the skin. The victim may feel a tingling sensation. Reapply the bandage more loosely.

APPLYING A ROLLER BANDAGE

Follow these general rules when you are applying a roller bandage:

- Keep the rolled part of the bandage (the head) uppermost as you work (the unrolled part is called the tail).
- Position yourself toward the front of the victim, on the injured side.
- Make sure that the injured part is supported in the position in which it will remain after bandaging.

> **ⓘ CAUTION**
>
> Once you have applied the bandage, check the circulation in the limb beyond it (opposite). This is especially important if you are applying an elasticized or gauze bandage because these mold to the shape of the limb and may become tighter if the limb swells.

1 Place the tail of the bandage below the injury. Bandaging from the inside of the limb outward, make two straight turns to anchor the tail in place.

Keep injured part supported while you work

Site of injury

Anchor tail

2 Make a series of spiraling turns with the bandage. Wind it from the inside to the outside of the upper surface of the limb, working upward. Each new turn should cover between one-half and two-thirds of the previous turn of bandaging.

Keep head of bandage uppermost

3 Finish with one straight turn, and secure the end of the bandage. If the bandage is too short, apply another one so that the injured area is covered.

Make straight turn to finish

4 As soon as you have finished, check the circulation beyond the bandage (opposite). If necessary, unroll the bandage until the blood supply returns, and reapply it more loosely.

Press and release nail to check circulation

TRIANGULAR BANDAGES

This type of bandage may be supplied as part of a first-aid kit. To make one, cut or fold a square yard of sturdy fabric diagonally in half. The bandage can be used in the following ways:

• Folded into a binder bandage (below) to immobilize and support a limb or to secure a splint or dressing.

• Folded into a cravat bandage

(below) to immobilize feet and ankles or hold a dressing in place

• Opened to form a sling.

OPEN TRIANGULAR BANDAGE

MAKING A BINDER BANDAGE

1 Open a triangular bandage and lay it flat on a clean surface. Fold it in half horizontally, so that the point of the triangle touches the center of the base.

2 Fold the triangular bandage in half again, in the same direction, so that the first folded edge touches the base. The bandage should now form a broad strip.

First folded edge aligned with base

End | Point | Base

MAKING A CRAVAT BANDAGE

1 Fold a triangular bandage to make a binder bandage (above).

2 Fold the bandage horizontally in half again. It should form a long, narrow, strip of material.

SQUARE KNOTS

Always use a square knot to secure a triangular bandage. It will not slip, it is easy to untie, and it lies flat, so it is more comfortable for the victim. Avoid tying the knot around or directly over the injury itself.

TYING A SQUARE KNOT

1 Pass the left end (dark) over and under the right end (light).

2 Lift both ends of the bandage above the rest of the material.

3 Pass the right end (dark) over and under the left end (light).

4 Pull the ends to tighten the knot, then tuck them under the bandage.

ARM SLING

An arm sling holds the forearm in a horizontal or slightly raised position. It provides support for an injured upper arm, wrist, or forearm, and is used for a victim whose elbow can be bent. An elevation sling (p.18) is used to keep the forearm and hand raised in a higher position.

1 Make sure that the injured arm is supported with its hand slightly raised. Fold the base of the bandage under to form a hem. Place the bandage with the base parallel to the victim's body and level with her little finger nail. Pass the upper end under the injured arm and then pull it around the neck to the opposite shoulder.

Pass end over shoulder and around back of neck

Hold point beyond elbow

2 Fold the lower end of the bandage up over the forearm and bring it to meet the upper end at the shoulder.

Upper end

Lower end of bandage

Point

3 Tie a square knot (opposite) on the injured side, at the hollow above the victim's collar bone. Tuck both free ends of the bandage under the knot to pad it.

Tie knot just above collar bone

Ensure sling supports forearm and hand up to little finger

4 Fold the point forward at the victim's elbow. Tuck loose fabric around the elbow, and secure the point to the front with a safety pin. If you do not have a pin, twist the point until the fabric fits the elbow snugly, then tuck it into the sling at the back of the arm.

SECURED WITHOUT PIN

Pin point at front of elbow

5 As soon as you have finished, check the circulation in the fingers (p.14). Recheck every 10 minutes. If necessary, loosen and reapply the bandages and sling.

ELEVATION SLING

This type of sling supports the forearm and hand in a raised position, with the fingertips touching the victim's shoulder. The elevation sling is used to help control bleeding from wounds in the forearm or hand, and minimize the swelling that often occurs as a result of burn injuries.

1 Ask the victim to support his injured arm across his chest, with the fingers resting on the opposite shoulder.

Ask victim to support his elbow

2 Place the bandage over his body, with one end over the uninjured shoulder. Hold the point just beyond his elbow.

Base of bandage

Hold point beyond elbow of injured side

3 Ask the victim to let go of his injured arm. Tuck the base of the bandage under his hand, forearm, and elbow.

Support arm as you work

Leave thumb showing

4 Bring the lower end of the bandage up diagonally across his back, to meet the other end at his shoulder.

Bring ends together

Pass lower end of bandage up across back

5 Tie the ends in a square knot (p.16) at the hollow above the victim's collar bone. Tuck the ends under the knot so that they pad it.

6 Twist the point until the bandage fits closely around the victim's elbow. Tuck the point in just above his elbow to secure it. If you have a safety pin, fold the fabric over the elbow, and fasten the point at the corner.

SECURED WITH PIN

Check thumb for signs of impaired circulation

Secure corner by twisting fabric and tucking it in

7 Regularly check the circulation in the thumb (p.14). If necessary, loosen and reapply the bandages and sling.

2

TO STAY ALIVE, we need an adequate supply of oxygen to enter our lungs and be transferred through the bloodstream to all cells in the body. If a victim is deprived of oxygen, the brain begins to fail. The victim will lose consciousness, the heartbeat and breathing will cease, and death results.

RESUSCITATION
To restore oxygen to the brain, the airway must be open so that oxygen can enter the body; breathing must be restored to enable oxygen to enter the bloodstream via the lungs; and blood must circulate to all tissues and organs. Therefore, the priority in treating an unconscious victim is to establish an open airway and maintain breathing and circulation. Since treatment is different for children and infants, this chapter gives separate step-by-step instructions for adults, children, and infants. Techniques for treating a choking victim are also given in this chapter.

✚ FIRST-AID PRIORITIES

● Maintain an open airway, check breathing, and resuscitate.
● If victim is choking, relieve airway obstruction if possible.

CONTENTS

LIFE-SAVING PROCEDURES

LIFE-SAVING PRIORITIES

With an unconscious victim, your priorities are:

• *To maintain an open airway*
An unconscious victim may lose muscular control, so the tongue may fall back and block the airway. Lifting the chin and tilting the head back lifts the tongue from the entrance of the air passage, thereby allowing the victim to breathe.

• *To breathe for the victim.* By giving rescue breaths you can force air into the victim's air passages and thus get oxygen into the bloodstream and circulating around the body.

• *To maintain blood circulation.* Chest compressions can be used to artificially maintain blood circulation and thus get oxygen-rich blood to the tissues. To make sure that the blood is adequately supplied with oxygen, chest compressions must always be combined with rescue breathing (together known as cardiopulmonary resuscitation or CPR).

In addition, a machine called a defibrillator can deliver a controlled electric shock that can restore a normal heartbeat.

The following factors increase the chances of survival if all elements are completed properly:

• Help is called quickly.
• Blood circulation is maintained by CPR.
• In an adult victim with no signs of circulation, a defibrillator is used promptly.
• The victim reaches the hospital quickly for specialized treatment.

Chain of survival
Four elements increase the chances of a collapsed adult victim surviving. If any one of the elements in this chain is missing, the chances are reduced.

Early help	Early CPR	Early defibrillation	Early advanced care
Dial 9·1·1 or call your local EMS so that a defibrillator and expert help arrive as quickly as possible.	Use chest compressions and rescue breaths to "buy time" until expert help arrives.	Give the victim a controlled electric shock. This jolts the heart into a normal rhythm.	Specialized treatment by EMTs and in the hospital quickly stabilizes the victim's condition.

WHEN TO CALL AN AMBULANCE

If you have a helper, send him to dial 9·1·1 or call EMS as soon as you know that the victim is not breathing. If you are on your own, your actions depend on the age of the victim and the likely cause of the unconsciousness.

CHILD OR INFANT VICTIM
Unconsciousness in an infant or child under 8 years is most likely to be due to a breathing problem. For this reason, you should give rescue breaths and chest compressions for 1 minute before leaving the child to dial 9·1·1.

ADULT VICTIM
If an adult victim is not breathing, and unconsciousness is due either to a heart problem, or an unknown cause, call 9·1·1 immediately. If unconsciousness is due to injury, drowning, or choking, give chest compressions and rescue breaths for 1 minute, then call 9·1·1.

ADULT RESUSCITATION CHART

The sequence below summarizes the main actions for dealing with an adult, or a child aged 8 or over, who is unconscious. The chart assumes that you have checked for any danger to yourself or the victim. The pages that follow give full details on each step in the resuscitation sequence.

CHECK VICTIM'S RESPONSE
- Try to get a response by asking questions and gently shaking his shoulders (p.22).
- Is there a response?

YES → Leave the victim in the position found, and summon help if needed.

NO

OPEN THE AIRWAY; CHECK FOR BREATHING
- Tilt the head back to open the airway (p.23), removing any obvious obstruction. Check for breathing (p.23).
- Is he breathing?

YES → Check for life-threatening injuries. Place the victim in the recovery position (pp.30–31), and then summon help.

NO

Send a helper to **DIAL 9·1·1 OR CALL EMS**

BREATHE FOR VICTIM
- Give two effective rescue breaths (pp.24–25).

NO

ASSESS FOR CIRCULATION
- Check for signs of circulation for not more than 10 seconds (p.26).
- Are there signs of circulation?

NO

COMMENCE CPR
- Alternate 15 chest compressions with two rescue breaths (pp.26–27).
- Repeat as necessary.

⊘ WARNING

If you are alone, dial 9·1·1 or call EMS as soon as you know the victim is not breathing – unless it is due to injury, choking, or drowning. In these cases, first give chest compressions and rescue breaths for 1 minute before calling (see WHEN TO CALL AN AMBULANCE, opposite).

YES → Continue giving rescue breaths. Check for signs of circulation after every minute (about 10 breaths). If the victim starts breathing but remains unconscious, place him in the recovery position (pp.30–31).

UNCONSCIOUS ADULT

The following pages give instructions for all the techniques needed in the resuscitation of an unconscious adult.

Always approach the victim from the side, kneeling next to his head or chest. You will then be in the correct position for all the possible stages of resuscitation: opening the victim's airway; checking breathing and circulation; and giving rescue breaths and chest compressions (called CPR or cardiopulmonary resuscitation).

At each stage, you will have decisions to make. The steps given here tell you what to do next in each situation.

The first priority is to open the airway so that the victim can breathe or you can give effective rescue breaths. If breathing and circulation return at any stage, place the victim in the recovery position. If there is no breathing or signs of circulation, a defibrillator, correctly used, will increase the chance of survival.

HOW TO CHECK RESPONSE

On discovering a collapsed victim, you should first establish whether he is conscious or unconscious. Do this by gently shaking the victim's shoulders. Ask "What has happened?" or give a command: "Open your eyes." Speak loudly and clearly.

> **❶ CAUTION**
>
> Always assume that there is a neck injury and shake the shoulders very gently.

Gently shake shoulders

IF THERE IS A RESPONSE

1 If there is no further danger, leave the victim in the position in which you found him and summon help if needed.

2 Treat any condition found and monitor vital signs – level of response, pulse, and breathing (pp.8–9).

3 Continue monitoring the victim until either help arrives or he recovers.

IF THERE IS NO RESPONSE

1 Shout for help. If possible, leave the victim in the position in which he was found and open the airway.

2 If this is not possible, turn him onto his back and open the airway.

▶ Go to HOW TO OPEN THE AIRWAY opposite

HOW TO OPEN THE AIRWAY

1 Kneel by the victim's head. Place one hand on his forehead. Gently tilt his head back. The mouth will fall open.

Hand on forehead tilts head back

3 Place the fingertips of your other hand under the point of the victim's chin and lift the chin.

Use fingertips to lift chin

2 Pick out obvious obstructions, such as dislodged dentures or broken teeth, from the victim's mouth. Do not do a finger sweep. Leave well-fitted dentures in place.

4 Check to see if the victim is now breathing.

Go to HOW TO CHECK BREATHING below

HOW TO CHECK BREATHING

Keeping the airway open, look, listen, and feel for breathing: look for chest movement, listen for sounds of breathing, and feel for breath on your cheek. Wait no more than 10 seconds before deciding breathing is absent.

Look along chest for movement indicating breathing

IF VICTIM IS BREATHING

1 Check the victim for any life-threatening injuries, such as severe bleeding, and treat as necessary.

2 Place the victim in the recovery position. Monitor vital signs – response, pulse, and breathing (pp.8–9).

Go to HOW TO PLACE IN RECOVERY POSITION, pp.30–31

IF VICTIM IS NOT BREATHING

1 DIAL 9·1·1 OR CALL EMS Send a helper to call if available. If you are alone, *see* WHEN TO CALL AN AMBULANCE, p.20.

2 Give two effective rescue breaths and then check for signs of circulation.

Go to HOW TO GIVE RESCUE BREATHS, pp.24–25

UNCONSCIOUS ADULT (continued)

HOW TO GIVE RESCUE BREATHS

1 Make sure that the victim's airway is still open by keeping one hand on his forehead and two fingers of the other hand under the tip of his chin.

Keep chin lifted so that airway is open

2 Move the hand that was on the forehead down to the nose. Pinch the soft part of the nose with the finger and thumb. Open the victim's mouth.

3 If you have a face shield or pocket mask (below), place it over the victim's mouth. Take a deep breath to fill your lungs with air and place your lips around the victim's mouth, making sure you make a good seal.

Continue to pinch the nose while taking a breath

SPECIAL CASE

USING A FACE SHIELD OR POCKET MASK
First aiders may receive training in the use of these aids. Face shields are plastic barriers with a reinforced hole to fit over the victim's mouth. The mask is more substantial and has a valve.

   If you are trained to use one of these aids, carry it with you at all times and use it if you need to resuscitate a victim. If you do not have a mask or shield, do not hesitate to give rescue breaths.

USING A FACE SHIELD

USING A POCKET MASK

---

4 Blow steadily into the victim's mouth until the chest rises. This usually takes about 2 seconds.

5 Maintaining head tilt and chin lift, remove your mouth and see if the victim's chest falls. If it rises visibly as you blow and falls fully when you lift your mouth away, you have given an effective breath. Give two effective breaths, then check for circulation.

▶ Go to HOW TO CHECK FOR CIRCULATION p.26

Watch the chest fall

IF YOU CANNOT ACHIEVE EFFECTIVE BREATHS

• Recheck the head tilt and chin lift.
• Recheck the victim's mouth. Remove any obvious obstructions, but do not do a finger sweep of the mouth.
• Make no more than five attempts to achieve two effective breaths.

If you still cannot achieve two effective breaths after five attempts, check the victim for signs of circulation.

▶ Go to HOW TO CHECK FOR CIRCULATION p.26

> **⚠ WARNING**
>
> If you know that the victim has choked, and you cannot achieve effective breaths, immediately begin giving chest compressions and rescue breaths to try to relieve the obstruction quickly (see HOW TO GIVE CPR, pp.26–27).

> **SPECIAL CASE**
>
> MOUTH-TO-NOSE RESCUE BREATHING
> In situations such as rescue from water or where injuries to the mouth make it impossible to achieve a good mouth-to-mouth seal, use the mouth-to-nose method for giving rescue breaths. With the victim's mouth closed, form a tight seal with your lips around the nose and blow steadily into the victim's nose. Then allow the mouth to fall open to let the air escape.

Make a tight seal around the nose

> **SPECIAL CASE**
>
> MOUTH-TO-STOMA RESCUE BREATHING
> A victim who has had the voice-box surgically removed breathes through a stoma (opening) in the front of the neck rather than the mouth and nose. Always check for a stoma before giving rescue breaths. If you find a stoma, close off the mouth and nose with your thumb and fingers and then breathe into the stoma.

Close off victim's mouth and nose with your thumb and fingers

UNCONSCIOUS ADULT (continued)

HOW TO CHECK FOR CIRCULATION

Still kneeling beside the victim's head, look, listen, and feel for signs of circulation, such as breathing, coughing, or movement. Check for signs of circulation for no more than 10 seconds.

IF THERE ARE NO SIGNS OF CIRCULATION
Begin giving chest compressions with rescue breaths immediately.

▶ Go to HOW TO GIVE CPR below

IF YOU ARE SURE YOU HAVE DETECTED SIGNS OF CIRCULATION

1 Continue rescue breathing. After every 10 breaths (about 1 minute), recheck for signs of circulation. If the victim starts to breathe but remains unconscious, place him in the recovery position (pp.30–31).

2 Monitor vital signs – level of response, pulse, and breathing (pp.8–9). Be prepared to turn the victim onto his back again to restart rescue breathing (pp.24–25).

Look and listen for breathing

HOW TO GIVE CPR

1 Kneel beside the victim. Remove or cut through upper-body clothing if possible. With the index and middle fingers of your lower hand, locate his lowermost rib on the side closer to you. Slide your fingertips along the rib to where it meets the breastbone. Place your middle finger at this point and your index finger beside it on the lower breastbone.

Kneel beside victim

Slide fingers up from lowermost rib

2 Place the heel of your other hand on the breastbone, and slide it down until it reaches your index finger. This is the point at which you should apply pressure.

Slide heel of hand down to meet fingers

3 Place the heel of your first hand on top of the other hand, and interlock your fingers.

Keep fingers clear of chest

4 Leaning well over the victim with your arms straight, press down vertically on the breastbone and depress the chest by about 1½–2 in (4–5 cm). Release the pressure without removing your hands from his chest.

5 Compress the chest 15 times at a rate of 100 compressions per minute. The time taken for compression and release should be about the same.

6 Tilt the head, lift the chin, and give two rescue breaths (pp.24–25).

Keep chin lifted to maintain the airway

7 Continue this cycle of alternating 15 chest compressions with two rescue breaths until emergency help arrives and takes over; the victim makes a movement or takes a spontaneous breath; or you become so exhausted that you cannot carry on.

Interlock fingers

Keep arms straight

Press straight down on heels of hands

UNCONSCIOUS ADULT (continued)

HOW TO USE A DEFIBRILLATOR

When the heart stops and there are no signs of circulation, a cardiac arrest has occurred. The most common cause is an abnormal heart rhythm, known as ventricular fibrillation. This can be caused by a heart attack or when the heart has insufficient oxygen. The rhythm can be corrected with a defibrillator (automated external defibrillator, or AED). These devices are available in many public places, including airports, and some shopping centers. A defibrillator analyzes the victim's heart rhythm and tells you what action to take at each stage. However, you must be trained in its use and be able to carry out CPR (pp.26–27).

You will probably have already started the life-saving sequence when the defibrillator arrives. Stop what you are doing and start using it.

> **❶ CAUTION**
>
> • Make sure that no one is touching the victim because this will interfere with the defibrillator readings.
>
> • Do not turn off the defibrillator or remove the pads at any time, even if the victim appears to have recovered.

1 Switch on the defibrillator and check that the electrode leads are plugged in. Remove or cut through clothing covering the chest and quickly wipe away any sweat. Shave chest hair if it is excessive because it will prevent the pads from sticking to the skin.

2 Carefully remove the backing paper from the electrode pads and attach them to the victim's chest in the position indicated on the pads.

3 The defibrillator will start analyzing the heart rhythm: ensure no one is touching the victim. Follow the visual and/or spoken prompts (opposite). These will advise you when a shock is to be administered, when to check for signs of circulation (p.26), and when to give chest compressions and rescue breaths (*see* HOW TO GIVE CPR, pp.26–27).

4 Continue to follow the prompts from the defibrillator until the emergency services arrive and advanced care is available. If at any time the victim starts breathing, place him in the recovery position (pp.30–31). Leave the defibrillator attached.

Make sure helper does not touch victim while machine is analyzing

Defibrillator

Place electrode pads on each side of heart

28

SEQUENCE OF DEFIBRILLATOR INSTRUCTIONS

The defibrillator will give a series of visual and verbal prompts as soon as it is switched on. Some older machines may tell you to check the pulse. In this case, check for signs of circulation; do not waste time trying to find the pulse. Continue to follow the prompts given by the defibrillator until emergency medical technicians arrive and advanced care is available.

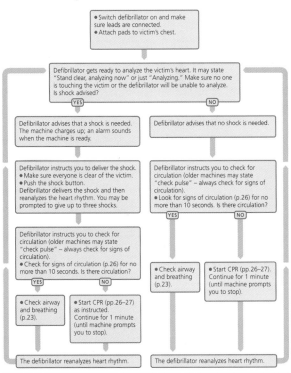

- Switch defibrillator on and make sure leads are connected.
- Attach pads to victim's chest.

Defibrillator gets ready to analyze the victim's heart. It may state "Stand clear, analyzing now" or just "Analyzing." Make sure no one is touching the victim or the defibrillator will be unable to analyze. Is shock advised?

YES

Defibrillator advises that a shock is needed. The machine charges up; an alarm sounds when the machine is ready.

Defibrillator instructs you to deliver the shock.
- Make sure everyone is clear of the victim.
- Push the shock button.
Defibrillator delivers the shock and then reanalyzes the heart rhythm. You may be prompted to give up to three shocks.

Defibrillator instructs you to check for circulation (older machines may state "check pulse" – always check for signs of circulation).
- Check for signs of circulation (p.26) for no more than 10 seconds. Is there circulation?

YES
- Check airway and breathing (p.23).

NO
- Start CPR (pp.26–27) as instructed. Continue for 1 minute (until machine prompts you to stop).

The defibrillator reanalyzes heart rhythm.

NO

Defibrillator advises that no shock is needed.

Defibrillator instructs you to check for circulation (older machines may state "check pulse" – always check for signs of circulation).
- Look for signs of circulation (p.26) for no more than 10 seconds. Is there circulation?

YES
- Check airway and breathing (p.23).

NO
- Start CPR (pp.26–27). Continue for 1 minute (until machine prompts you to stop).

The defibrillator reanalyzes heart rhythm.

UNCONSCIOUS ADULT (continued)

HOW TO PLACE IN RECOVERY POSITION

1 Kneel beside the victim. Remove eyeglasses and any very bulky objects, such as cellular phones and large bunches of keys, from the pockets. Do not search the pockets for small items.

2 Make sure that both of the victim's legs are straight.

3 Place the arm that is closer to you at a right angle to the victim's body, with the elbow bent and the palm of the hand facing upward.

❗ WARNING

If you suspect a spinal injury, leave the victim in the position in which he was found, and maintain an open airway by using the jaw thrust method (p.81). If the victim must be moved to open the airway, use the log-roll technique (p.81).

❗ CAUTION

If the victim is found lying on his side or front, not all these steps will be necessary to place him in the recovery position.

Make sure that legs are straight

Place arm at right angle to the body

4 Bring the arm that is farther from you across the victim's chest, and hold the back of his hand against the cheek nearer to you. With your other hand, grasp the far leg just above the knee and pull it up, keeping the foot flat on the ground.

Foot is flat on ground

Hold victim's hand, palm outward, against his cheek

5 Keeping the victim's hand pressed against his cheek, pull on the far leg and roll the victim toward you and onto his side.

Hold onto victim's leg and pull it over

6 Adjust the upper leg so that both the hip and the knee are bent at right angles.

Bent leg props up body and prevents victim from rolling forward

Hand under cheek helps to keep airway open

7 Tilt the victim's head back so that the airway remains open. If necessary, adjust the hand under the cheek to make sure that the head remains tilted and the airway stays open.

8 If it has not already been done, DIAL 9·1·1 OR CALL EMS Monitor and record vital signs – level of response, pulse, and breathing (pp.8–9).

9 If the victim has to be left in the recovery position for longer than 30 minutes, roll him onto his back, and then onto the opposite side periodically unless other injuries prevent this.

SPECIAL CASE

USING TWO OR MORE RESCUERS
Unless you saw the victim collapse, you may not know for sure whether he could have injured his back when he fell. Therefore, if you have one or more helpers, it is best to work together to place the victim in the recovery position.

• If you have a helper, one of you should steady the head and neck while the other turns the victim (right).

• With three people, one person steadies the head and neck while one person turns the victim. The third person should keep the victim's back straight during the maneuver.

• If there are four or more people in total available to help, use the log-roll technique (p.81).

CHILD RESUSCITATION CHART

The resuscitation method depends on the child's age and size. In children aged 1–7, respiratory failure (absence of breathing) is the main reason for the heart to stop. Ask a helper to dial 9·1·1 or call EMS while you treat the child; if you are alone, resuscitate for 1 minute before calling.

For a child aged 8 or over, use adult resuscitation methods (pp.21–31).

CHECK CHILD'S RESPONSE
- Try to get a response by asking questions and gently tapping the child's shoulder.
- Is there a response?

`YES` → Leave the child in the position found and summon help if needed.

`NO`

OPEN THE AIRWAY; CHECK FOR BREATHING
- Assuming no neck injury, tilt the head back (p.34), and remove obvious obstructions. Check for breathing (p.34).
- Is the child breathing?

`YES` → Check for life-threatening injuries. Place the child in the recovery position (pp.38–39) and summon help.

`NO`

Send a helper to DIAL 9·1·1 OR CALL EMS

BREATHE FOR CHILD
- Give two effective rescue breaths (p.35).

`NO`

❶ WARNING

If you are alone, carry out rescue breathing and chest compressions for 1 minute before leaving the child to call for help (*see* WHEN TO CALL AN AMBULANCE, p.20).

ASSESS FOR CIRCULATION
- Check for signs of circulation for no more than 10 seconds (p.36).
- Are there signs of circulation?

`NO`

`YES` → Continue rescue breathing. After every 20 breaths (about 1 minute), recheck for signs of circulation. If the child starts to breathe but remains unconscious, place her in the recovery position (pp.38–39).

COMMENCE CPR
- Alternate five chest compressions with one rescue breath (pp.36–37).
- Repeat as necessary.

UNCONSCIOUS CHILD (1–7 years)

The following pages give instructions for resuscitating a child who collapses. For a child aged 8 or over, use the adult method (pp.21–31).

Always approach the child from the side, kneeling next to the head or chest. You will then be in the correct position for all the possible stages of resuscitation: opening the airway, checking the breathing and circulation, and giving rescue breaths and chest compressions (called CPR or cardiopulmonary resuscitation).

The steps given here will guide you through each technique, then advise you on what to do next. Your first priority is to ensure that the airway is clear so that the child can breathe or you can give effective rescue breaths if needed. If normal breathing and circulation resume, place the child in the recovery position (pp.38–39).

Dial 9·1·1 or call EMS immediately if a child who has a known heart disease collapses, because early access to advanced care may be life-saving.

HOW TO CHECK FOR RESPONSE

On discovering a collapsed child, you should first establish whether she is conscious or unconscious. Do this by speaking loudly and clearly to the child. Ask "What has happened?" or give a command: "Open your eyes." Place one hand on her shoulder, and gently tap her.

Gently tap shoulder

IF THERE IS A RESPONSE

1 If there is no further danger, leave the child in the position in which she was found and summon help if needed.

2 Treat any condition found. Regularly monitor vital signs – level of response, pulse, and breathing (pp.8–9).

3 Continue this until either help arrives or the child recovers.

IF THERE IS NO RESPONSE

1 Shout for help. If possible, leave the child in the position in which you found her, then open the airway.

2 If this is not possible, turn the child onto her back and open the airway.

▶ Go to HOW TO OPEN THE AIRWAY p.34

UNCONSCIOUS CHILD (continued)

HOW TO OPEN THE AIRWAY

1 Kneel by the child's head. If there is no neck injury, place one hand on her forehead and gently tilt her head back. The mouth will fall open.

2 With your fingertips, pick out any obvious obstructions from the mouth. Do not do a finger sweep.

Use fingertips only to remove obstruction

3 Place the fingertips of your other hand under the point of the child's chin and gently lift the chin.

Place two fingers under chin

4 Check to see whether the child is now breathing.

▶ Go to HOW TO CHECK BREATHING below

HOW TO CHECK BREATHING

Keep the airway open and look, listen, and feel for breathing – look for chest movement, listen for sounds of breathing, and feel for breath on your cheek. Do this for no more than 10 seconds.

Lean right down over victim

Look for chest movement, indicating breathing

IF THE CHILD IS BREATHING

1 Check for any life-threatening injuries such as severe bleeding. Treat as necessary.

2 Place the child in the recovery position. Regularly monitor her vital signs – level of response, pulse, and breathing (pp.8–9).

▶ Go to HOW TO PLACE IN THE RECOVERY POSITION pp.38–39

IF THE CHILD IS NOT BREATHING

1 Ask a helper to DIAL 9·1·1 OR CALL EMS

2 Give two effective rescue breaths (right) and then check the child for signs of circulation.

▶ Go to HOW TO GIVE RESCUE BREATHS opposite

HOW TO GIVE RESCUE BREATHS

1 Ensure that the airway is still open by keeping one hand on the child's forehead and two fingers of the other hand under her chin.

Tilt head gently

2 Pinch the soft part of the child's nose with the finger and thumb of the hand that was on the forehead. Make sure that her nostrils are closed to prevent air from escaping. Open her mouth.

Keep chin lifted

3 Take a deep breath to fill your lungs with air. Place your lips around the child's mouth, making sure that you form an airtight seal.

Make sure nostrils are tightly closed

4 Blow steadily into the child's mouth until her chest rises.

5 Maintaining head tilt and chin lift, take your mouth off the child's mouth and see if her chest falls. If the chest rises visibly as you blow and falls fully when you lift your mouth, you have given an effective breath. Give two effective breaths, then check for signs of circulation.

▶ Go to HOW TO CHECK FOR CIRCULATION p.36

Watch chest fall

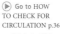

IF YOU CANNOT ACHIEVE EFFECTIVE BREATHS

- Recheck the head tilt and chin lift.
- Recheck the child's mouth. Remove any obvious obstructions, but do not do a finger sweep of the mouth.
- Make no more than five attempts to achieve two effective breaths.

If you still cannot achieve two effective rescue breaths, check the child for signs of circulation.

▶ Go to HOW TO CHECK FOR CIRCULATION p.36

> **❶ WARNING**
>
> If you know that the child has choked, and you cannot achieve effective breaths, you must immediately begin giving chest compressions to try to relieve the obstruction quickly (*see* HOW TO GIVE CPR, pp.36–37).

UNCONSCIOUS CHILD (continued)

HOW TO CHECK FOR CIRCULATION

Still kneeling beside the child's head, look, listen, and feel for signs of circulation, such as breathing, coughing, or movement. Check for these signs of circulation for no more than 10 seconds.

Look and listen for breathing

IF THERE ARE NO SIGNS OF CIRCULATION

Begin chest compressions and rescue breaths (cardiopulmonary resuscitation – CPR) immediately. Continue this for 1 minute then DIAL 9·1·1 OR CALL EMS

▶ Go to HOW TO GIVE CPR below

IF YOU ARE SURE YOU HAVE DETECTED SIGNS OF CIRCULATION

1 Continue rescue breathing for 1 minute. Then DIAL 9·1·1 OR CALL EMS. After every 20 breaths (about 1 minute), check for signs of circulation. If the child starts to breathe but remains unconscious, place her in the recovery position (pp.38–39).

2 Monitor and record vital signs – level of response, pulse, and breathing (pp.8–9). Be prepared to turn the child onto her back again to restart rescue breathing (p.35).

HOW TO GIVE CPR

1 Kneel beside the child, and remove her shirt if possible. With the fingertips of your lower hand, locate one of her lowermost ribs on the side nearer to you. Slide your fingertips along the rib to the point where the lowermost ribs meet at the breastbone. Place your middle finger at this point and your index finger beside it on the lower breastbone.

Kneel beside victim

Slide fingers up from lowermost rib

2 Place the heel of your other hand on the breastbone and slide it down until it reaches your index finger. This is the point at which you will apply pressure.

Slide heel of hand down to meet fingers

3 Use the heel of one hand only to apply pressure – keep your fingers raised so that you do not apply pressure to the child's ribs.

Keep fingers clear of chest

4 Leaning well over the child, with your arm straight, press down vertically on the breastbone, depressing the chest by one-third of its depth. Release the pressure without removing your hand.

5 Compress the chest five times, at a rate of 100 compressions per minute. Compression and release should take the same amount of time.

6 Tilt the head, lift the chin, and give one rescue breath (p.35).

Keep chin lifted to maintain the airway

7 Continue this cycle of alternating five chest compressions with one rescue breath until emergency help arrives and takes over; the child makes a movement or takes a spontaneous breath; or you become so exhausted that you cannot continue.

Keep arm straight

Press straight down with heel of hand

UNCONSCIOUS CHILD (continued)

HOW TO PLACE IN RECOVERY POSITION

1 Kneel beside the child. Remove any eyeglasses and very bulky objects from the pockets, but do not search for small items.

2 Make sure that both of the child's legs are straight. Place the arm that is closer to you at a right angle to the child's body, with the elbow bent and the palm facing upward.

> **❶ WARNING**
>
> If you suspect a spinal injury, maintain an open airway with the child in the position in which she was found and by using the jaw thrust method (p.81). If the victim must be moved in order to open the airway, use the log-roll technique (p.81).

Straighten legs

Place arm at right angle to the body

3 Bring the arm that is farther away from you across the child's chest, and hold the back of her hand against the cheek nearer you. With your other hand, grasp the far leg just above the knee and pull it up, keeping the foot flat on the ground.

Foot flat on ground

Hold child's hand, palm outward, against her cheek

> **❶ CAUTION**
>
> If the child is found lying on her side or front, not all of these steps will be necessary to place her in the recovery position.

4 Keeping the child's hand pressed against her cheek, pull on the far leg and roll the child toward you and onto her side.

Tilt chin so that fluid can drain from mouth

Pull bent leg toward you

5 Adjust the upper leg so that both the hip and the knee are bent at right angles. Tilt the child's head back so that the airway remains open. If necessary, adjust the hand under the cheek to make sure that the head remains tilted and the airway stays open.

Hand supports head

Bent leg props up body and prevents child from rolling forward

Make sure that head is tilted well back

6 If it has not already been done, DIAL 9·1·1 OR CALL EMS Monitor and record her vital signs – level of response, pulse, and breathing (pp.8–9) – until medical help arrives.

7 If the child has to be left in the recovery position for longer than 30 minutes, roll her onto her back, then turn her onto the opposite side periodically – unless her other injuries prevent you from doing this.

SPECIAL CASE

USING TWO OR MORE RESCUERS
Unless you saw the child collapse, you may not know for sure whether she could have injured her back when she fell. If you have any helpers, you can work together to place the victim in the recovery position.
• If you have a helper, one of you should steady the head and neck while the other turns the victim (p.31, box).
• With three people, one person steadies the head and neck while another turns the victim. The third person should keep the victim's back straight during the maneuver.
• If there are four or more people in total who are available to help, use the log-roll technique (p.81).

INFANT RESUSCITATION CHART

In infants under 1 year, a breathing problem is the most probable reason for the heart to stop. As soon as you have established that the infant is not breathing, ask a helper to dial 9·1·1 or call EMS while you treat the infant.

CHECK INFANT'S RESPONSE
• Gently tap or flick the sole of the infant's foot. Never shake an infant.
• Is there a response?

YES → Take the infant with you to summon help if needed.

NO

OPEN THE AIRWAY; CHECK FOR BREATHING
• Place one hand on the infant's forehead and very gently tilt the head back. Remove any obvious obstruction. Lift the chin. Check for breathing (p.42).
• Is the infant breathing?

YES → Check for life-threatening injuries. Hold the infant in the recovery position (p.44) and summon help.

NO

Send a helper to DIAL 9·1·1 OR CALL EMS

BREATHE FOR INFANT
• Give two effective rescue breaths (pp.42–43).

NO

⊘ WARNING

If you are alone, do rescue breathing and chest compressions for 1 minute before taking the infant with you to dial 9·1·1 or call EMS (see WHEN TO CALL AN AMBULANCE, p.20).

ASSESS FOR CIRCULATION
• Check for signs of circulation for no more than 10 seconds (p.43).
• Are there signs of circulation?

YES → Continue rescue breathing. After every 20 breaths (about 1 minute) recheck for signs of circulation. If the infant starts to breathe but remains unconscious, hold him in the recovery position (p.44).

NO

COMMENCE CPR
• Alternate five chest compressions with one rescue breath (p.44).
• Repeat as necessary.

UNCONSCIOUS INFANT (under 1 year)

The following pages give instructions for resuscitating an infant under 1 year who is apparently lifeless. (For treating an older child see pp.32–39.)

Always treat the infant from the side. You will then be in the correct position for all the possible stages of resuscitation.

The steps here guide you through each technique. Your first priority is to make sure that the airway is open and clear. If breathing and circulation resume, hold the infant in the recovery position (p.44). Dial 9·1·1 or call EMS immediately if an infant has known heart disease.

HOW TO CHECK FOR RESPONSE

Gently tap or flick the sole of the infant's foot and call his name to see if he responds. Never shake an infant.

IF THERE IS A RESPONSE
Take the infant with you to summon help if needed. Monitor vital signs – level of response, pulse, and breathing (pp.8–9) – until help arrives.

IF THERE IS NO RESPONSE
Shout for help, then open the airway.

▶ Go to HOW TO OPEN THE AIRWAY below

Tap or flick
sole of foot

HOW TO OPEN THE AIRWAY

1 Place a hand on the infant's forehead and very gently tilt the head back.

2 Pick out any obvious obstructions from the infant's mouth. Do not do a finger sweep.

3 Place one fingertip of the other hand under the point of the chin. Gently lift the chin. Do not push on the soft tissues under the chin as this may block the airway.

Use your
fingertips
to remove
obstructions

Use one finger
to tilt chin
gently

4 Check to see if the infant is now breathing.

▶ Go to HOW TO CHECK BREATHING p.42

UNCONSCIOUS INFANT (continued)

HOW TO CHECK FOR BREATHING

Keep the airway open and look, listen, and feel for breathing – look for chest movement, listen for sounds of breathing, and feel for breath on your cheek. Do this for no more than 10 seconds.

Lean right down over infant

Look for chest movement, which indicates breathing

IF THE INFANT IS BREATHING

1 Check the infant for life-threatening injuries, such as severe bleeding, and treat if necessary.

2 Hold the infant in the recovery position. Regularly monitor vital signs – level of response, pulse, and breathing (pp.8–9).

▶ Go to HOW TO HOLD IN RECOVERY POSITION p.44

IF THE INFANT IS NOT BREATHING

1 Ask a helper to DIAL 9·1·1 OR CALL EMS

2 Give two effective rescue breaths and then check for signs of circulation.

▶ Go to HOW TO GIVE RESCUE BREATHS below

HOW TO GIVE RESCUE BREATHS

1 Make sure that the airway is still open by keeping one hand on the infant's forehead and one fingertip of the other hand under the tip of his chin.

Use one finger to lift chin

2 Take a breath. Place your lips around the infant's mouth and nose to form an airtight seal. If you cannot make a seal around the mouth and nose, close the infant's mouth and make a seal around the nose only.

3 Blow steadily into the infant's lungs until the chest rises.

Blow until chest rises

4 Maintaining the head tilt and chin lift, take your mouth off the infant's face and see if the chest falls. If the chest rises visibly as you blow and falls fully when you lift your mouth away, you have given an effective breath.

Watch chest fall

5 Give another effective rescue breath and then check for circulation.

▶ Go to HOW TO CHECK FOR CIRCULATION below

IF YOU CANNOT ACHIEVE EFFECTIVE BREATHS

- Recheck the head tilt and chin lift.
- Recheck the infant's mouth. Remove any obvious obstructions, but do not do a finger sweep of the mouth.
- Check that you have a firm seal around the mouth and nose.
- Make no more than five attempts to achieve two effective breaths. If you still cannot achieve two effective breaths, check the infant for signs of circulation.

▶ Go to HOW TO CHECK FOR CIRCULATION below

❶ WARNING

If you know that the infant has choked, and you cannot achieve effective breaths, immediately start chest compressions to try to relieve the obstruction quickly (*see* HOW TO GIVE CPR, p.44).

HOW TO CHECK FOR CIRCULATION

Look, listen, and feel for signs of circulation, such as breathing, coughing, or movement. Check for these signs for no more than 10 seconds.

Look and listen for breathing

IF THERE ARE NO SIGNS OF CIRCULATION

Begin CPR immediately (p.44). Continue for 1 minute, then DIAL 9·1·1 OR CALL EMS

IF YOU ARE SURE YOU HAVE DETECTED SIGNS OF CIRCULATION

1 Continue rescue breaths for 1 minute, then DIAL 9·1·1 OR CALL EMS After every 20 breaths (about 1 minute), check for signs of circulation.

2 If the infant begins to breathe but remains unconscious, hold him in the recovery position.

▶ Go to HOW TO HOLD IN THE RECOVERY POSITION p.44

UNCONSCIOUS INFANT (continued)

HOW TO GIVE CPR

1 Place the infant on his back on a flat surface at about waist height, or on the floor. Remove his clothing. Place two fingertips of your lower hand one finger's width below an imaginary line joining the infant's nipples. Take care not to press on the tip of the breastbone or the abdomen.

2 Press down vertically on the infant's breastbone and depress the chest by one-third of its depth. Release the pressure without losing the contact between your fingers and the breastbone.

Press down firmly and rhythmically

3 Compress the chest five times, at a rate of 100 times per minute. Compression and release should take the same amount of time.

4 Maintaining head tilt and chin lift, give one rescue breath through the mouth and nose (pp.42–43), or just the nose if necessary.

5 Continue this cycle of alternating five chest compressions with one rescue breath until emergency services arrive and take over; the infant makes a movement or takes a spontaneous breath; or you become so exhausted that you cannot continue.

HOW TO HOLD IN RECOVERY POSITION

1 Cradle the infant in your arms with his head tilted downward. This position prevents him from choking on his tongue or inhaling vomit.

2 Monitor and record vital signs – level of response, pulse, and breathing (pp.8–9) – until help arrives.

CHOKING SUMMARY CHARTS

The following pages explain how to treat a choking adult, child, or infant. The charts below summarize how to treat choking in a conscious victim. In an adult or a child, always encourage coughing first, and start the procedures described when the victim shows signs of weakening.

⚠ WARNING

If at any stage the victim becomes unconscious, you should open the airway, check breathing, and, if necessary, begin rescue breaths. If you cannot achieve effective breaths, begin giving chest compressions immediately to try to relieve the obstruction quickly (p.26, p.36, p.44).

PROCEDURE FOR ADULT *see p.46*

If the victim can speak and breathe **ENCOURAGE HIM OR HER TO TRY TO COUGH UP THE OBSTRUCTION**

If the obstruction is still present or the victim is getting weaker **GIVE UP TO FIVE ABDOMINAL THRUSTS**
• Check the mouth and remove any obvious obstruction.

If the obstruction does not clear after three cycles of abdominal thrusts and checking the mouth **DIAL 9-1-1 OR CALL EMS** Continue until help arrives.

PROCEDURE FOR CHILD (1–7 years) *see p.47*

If the victim can speak and breathe **ENCOURAGE HIM OR HER TO TRY TO COUGH UP THE OBSTRUCTION**

If the obstruction is still present or the child is getting weaker **GIVE UP TO FIVE ABDOMINAL THRUSTS**
• Check the mouth; remove any obvious obstruction.

If the obstruction is still present **GIVE UP TO FIVE MORE ABDOMINAL THRUSTS**
• Check the mouth and remove any obvious obstruction.

If the obstruction does not clear after three cycles of chest thrusts and abdominal thrusts **DIAL 9-1-1 OR CALL EMS** Continue until help arrives.

PROCEDURE FOR INFANT (under 1 year) *see p.48*

GIVE UP TO FIVE BACK SLAPS
• Check the mouth and remove any obvious obstruction.

If the obstruction is still present **GIVE UP TO FIVE CHEST THRUSTS**
• Check the mouth; remove any obvious obstruction.

If the obstruction does not clear after three cycles of back slaps and chest thrusts **DIAL 9-1-1 OR CALL EMS** Continue until help arrives.

CHOKING ADULT

If blockage of the airway is partial, the victim should be able to clear it himself; if it is complete, he will be unable to speak, breathe, or cough, and will soon lose consciousness. Be prepared to begin rescue breaths and chest compressions immediately. The throat muscles may relax slightly, leaving the airway sufficiently open for rescue breathing.

RECOGNITION

With partial obstruction:
- Coughing and distress.
- Difficulty speaking.

With complete obstruction:
- Inability to speak, breathe, or cough, and eventual loss of consciousness.

▶ See also UNCONSCIOUS ADULT pp.21–31

➕ YOUR AIMS

- To remove the obstruction.
- To arrange urgent transportation to the hospital if necessary.

❶ WARNING

If the victim becomes unconscious, open his airway, check breathing, and give rescue breaths (pp.23–25). If you cannot achieve effective breaths, immediately begin giving chest compressions to try to relieve the obstruction quickly (see HOW TO GIVE CPR, pp.26–27).

1 If the victim is able to speak, breathe, or cough, encourage him to continue coughing to relieve the obstruction.

If he can cough, the victim should try to clear the obstruction himself

2 If the victim is becoming weak, or stops breathing or coughing, carry out abdominal thrusts. Stand behind the victim and put both arms around the upper part of the abdomen. Make sure that he is bending forward. Clench your fist and place it (thumb inward)

between the navel and the bottom of the breastbone. Grasp your fist with your other hand. Pull sharply inward and upward up to five times.

Make a fist with one hand, and position it with thumb side against the abdomen

3 Check his mouth. If the obstruction is still not cleared, repeat steps 2 and 3 up to three times, checking his mouth after each step.

4 If the obstruction still has not cleared, DIAL 9·1·1 OR CALL EMS Continue until help arrives or the victim becomes unconscious.

❶ WARNING

If the victim is pregnant or obese, or you cannot reach around the victim's abdomen, give chest thrusts instead of abdominal thrusts. Position your fist in the middle of the victim's chest, grab your fist with the other hand, and pull sharply inward up to five times.

CHOKING CHILD (1–7 years)

Young children are particularly prone to choking. A child may choke on food, or put objects into his mouth and cause a blockage of the airway. For this reason, you should make sure that none of your child's toys have small parts that could be removed and choked on if your child is too young to understand that this is a dangerous thing to do.

If a child is choking, you need to act quickly. If he loses consciousness, be prepared to begin rescue breaths

RECOGNITION

With partial obstruction:
- Coughing and distress.
- Difficulty speaking.

With complete obstruction:
- Inability to speak, breathe, or cough, and eventual loss of consciousness.

and chest compressions. The throat muscles may relax, leaving the airway sufficiently open for rescue breathing.

▶ See also UNCONSCIOUS CHILD pp.33–39

➕ YOUR AIMS

- To remove the obstruction.
- To arrange urgent transportation to the hospital if necessary.

1 If the child is breathing, encourage him to cough; this may be enough to clear the obstruction.

Encourage child to cough

⊘ WARNING

If at any stage the child becomes unconscious, open the airway, check breathing, and give rescue breaths (pp.34–35). If you cannot achieve effective breaths, you should immediately begin giving chest compressions to try to relieve the obstruction quickly (*see* HOW TO GIVE CPR, pp.36–37).

2 If the child shows signs of becoming weak, or stops breathing or coughing, carry out abdominal thrusts. Put your arms around the child's upper abdomen. Make sure that he is bending well forward. Place your fist between the navel and the bottom of the breastbone, and grasp it with your other hand. Pull sharply inward and upward up to five times. Stop if the obstruction clears. Check his mouth.

Make sure that child is bending well forward

Fist should be just above child's navel

3 If the obstruction is still not cleared, repeat step 2 up to three times.

4 If the obstruction still has not cleared, DIAL 9·1·1 OR CALL EMS Continue until help arrives or the child becomes unconscious.

CHOKING INFANT (under 1 year)

An infant may readily choke on food or small objects. He will rapidly become distressed, and you need to act fast. If he loses consciousness, be prepared to give rescue breaths and chest compressions. When he is unconscious, the throat muscles may relax, opening the airway for rescue breathing, and chest compressions may clear the obstruction.

> RECOGNITION

With partial obstruction:
- Coughing and distress.
- Difficulty crying or making any other noise.

With complete obstruction:
- Inability to breathe or cough, and eventual loss of consciousness.

▶ See also UNCONSCIOUS INFANT pp.41–44

➕ YOUR AIMS

- To remove the obstruction.
- To arrange urgent transportation to the hospital if necessary.

❗ WARNING

If the infant becomes unconscious, open the airway, check breathing, and give rescue breaths (pp.41–43). If you cannot achieve effective breaths, immediately begin chest compressions to try to relieve the obstruction quickly (*see* HOW TO GIVE CPR, p.44).

1 If the infant is distressed, shows signs of becoming weak, or stops breathing or coughing, lay him face down along your forearm, with his head low, and support his back and head. Give up to five back slaps.

Make sure that head is below level of chest

2 Check the infant's mouth; remove any obvious obstructions with your fingertips. Do not do a finger sweep of the mouth.

3 If this fails to clear the obstruction, turn the infant onto his back and give up to five chest thrusts. Using two fingers, push inward and upward (toward the head) against the infant's breastbone, one finger's width below the nipple line.

Push on breastbone with your fingertips, one finger's breadth below nipple line

4 Perform five chest thrusts, at a rate of one every 3 seconds. The aim is to relieve the obstruction with each chest thrust rather than necessarily doing all five. Check the mouth.

5 If the obstruction is not cleared, repeat steps 1–4 three times. If the obstruction still has not cleared, take the infant with you to
DIAL 9·1·1 OR CALL EMS
Continue until help arrives or the infant becomes unconscious.

3

CIRCULATORY AND RESPIRATORY PROBLEMS

THE HEART and the network of blood vessels, collectively known as the circulatory (cardiovascular) system, pump blood around the body, carrying oxygen and nutrients to all body tissues. The structures that enable us to breathe, or take in oxygen and expel carbon dioxide, make up the respiratory system.

WHAT CAN GO WRONG
The circulatory system may be disrupted in two main ways: severe bleeding and fluid loss may cause the volume of blood to fall, depriving the organs of oxygen; or age or disease may cause the system to break down. Respiration can be impaired in various ways: the airways may be blocked; the lungs may be affected by inhalation of smoke or fumes or impaired by chest injury; or breathing may be affected by conditions such as asthma.

✚ FIRST-AID PRIORITIES

- Assess the victim's condition.
- Comfort and reassure the victim.
- Maintain an open airway, check breathing, and be prepared to resuscitate if necessary.
- Obtain medical aid if necessary. Dial 9·1·1 or call EMS if you suspect a serious illness or injury.

SHOCK

This life-threatening condition requires immediate emergency treatment to prevent permanent organ damage and death. Shock can be made worse by fear and pain; where there is a risk of shock developing, reassuring the victim and making her comfortable may be sufficient to keep her condition from deteriorating.

CAUSES OF SHOCK

The most common cause of shock is severe blood loss. Such blood loss may result from wounds, bleeding from internal organs, blood escaping into a body cavity, or bleeding from damaged blood vessels due to a fracture (p.70).

Shock can also result from loss of other body fluids due to diarrhea, vomiting, blockage in the intestine, or severe burns. It may occur when the heart is unable to pump blood, possibly due to severe heart disease, heart attack, or acute heart failure.

Other causes of shock include overwhelming infection, lack of certain hormones, low blood sugar (hypoglycemia), hypothermia,

RECOGNITION

Initially:
- A rapid pulse.
- Pale, cold, clammy skin; sweating.

As shock develops:
- Gray–blue skin (cyanosis) is apparent, especially inside the lips. A fingernail or earlobe, if pressed, will not regain its color immediately.
- Weakness and dizziness.
- Nausea, and possibly vomiting.
- Thirst.
- Rapid, shallow breathing.
- A weak, "thready" pulse.

As the brain's oxygen supply weakens:
- Restlessness and aggressiveness.
- Yawning and gasping for air.
- Unconsciousness.

Finally, the heart will stop.

severe allergic reaction (anaphylactic shock), drug overdose, and injury to the spinal cord.

▶ See also ANAPHYLACTIC SHOCK p.52
- LIFE-SAVING PROCEDURES pp.19–48
- SEVERE BLEEDING pp.60–61
- SEVERE BURNS AND SCALDS pp.98–99

EFFECTS OF BLOOD OR FLUID LOSS

Approximate volume lost	Effects on the body
1 pint (about 0.5 liter)	Little or no effect; this is the quantity normally taken in a blood-donor session
Up to 4 pints (2 liters)	Hormones such as epinephrine are released, quickening the pulse and inducing sweating ● Small blood vessels in non-vital areas, such as the skin, shut down to divert blood and oxygen to the vital organs ● Shock becomes evident
4 pints (2 liters) or more (over a third of the normal volume in the average adult)	As blood or fluid loss approaches this level, the pulse at the wrist may become undetectable ● Victim will usually lose consciousness ● Breathing may cease and the heart may stop

+ YOUR AIMS

- To recognize shock.
- To treat any obvious cause of shock.
- To improve the blood supply to the brain, heart, and lungs.
- To arrange urgent removal to the hospital.

⊘ CAUTION

- Do not let the victim eat, drink, smoke, or move unnecessarily. If she complains of thirst, moisten her lips with a little water.
- Do not leave the victim unattended, except to call an ambulance.
- Do not try to warm the victim with a hot-water bottle or any other direct source of heat.

1 Treat any possible cause of shock that you can detect, such as severe bleeding (pp.60–61) or serious burns (p.98).

2 Lay the victim down on a blanket to insulate her from the cold ground. Constantly reassure her.

3 Raise and support her legs to improve the blood supply to the vital organs. Be careful if you suspect a fracture.

Raise victim's legs so that they are higher than her heart

Keeping head low may prevent victim losing consciousness

4 Loosen tight clothing at the neck, chest, and waist to reduce constriction in these areas.

5 Keep the victim warm by covering her body and legs with coats or blankets. DIAL 9·1·1 OR CALL EMS

6 Monitor and record vital signs – level of response, pulse, and breathing (pp.8–9). If the victim becomes unconscious, open her airway and check breathing; be prepared to give rescue breaths and chest compressions if necessary (see LIFE-SAVING PROCEDURES, pp.19–48).

Take pulse at wrist

Protect victim from cold with coats or blankets

ANAPHYLACTIC SHOCK

A severe and potentially fatal allergic reaction, anaphylactic shock may develop within seconds or minutes of contact with a trigger, including:
• Skin or airborne contact with particular materials.
• The injection of a specific drug.
• The sting of a certain insect.
• Ingestion of a food such as peanuts.
Chemicals released into the blood widen (dilate) blood vessels and constrict (narrow) air passages. Blood pressure falls, breathing is impaired, the tongue and throat may swell, and the vital organs are starved of oxygen.

RECOGNITION
• Anxiety.
• Widespread red, blotchy skin eruption.
• Swelling of the tongue and throat.
• Puffiness around the eyes.
• Impaired breathing, ranging from a tight chest to severe difficulty; the victim may wheeze and gasp for air.
• Signs of shock (pp.50–51).

A victim may need emergency treatment with an injection of epinephrine (adrenaline). Priorities are to ease breathing and minimize shock until specialized help arrives.

+ YOUR AIM
• To arrange urgent removal to the hospital.

! WARNING
If the victim becomes unconscious, open her airway and check breathing; be prepared to give rescue breaths and chest compressions if necessary (see LIFE-SAVING PROCEDURES, pp.19–48). If the victim is breathing, place her in the recovery position (pp.30–31).

1 DIAL 9·1·1 OR CALL EMS
Give any information you have on the cause of the victim's condition.

2 Check whether the victim has the necessary medication – a syringe or an auto-injector of epinephrine (adrenaline) for self-administration. Help her to use it. If the victim is unable to administer the medication, and you have been trained to use an auto-injector, give it to her yourself.

3 If the victim is conscious, help her sit up in the position that most relieves any breathing difficulty.

4 Treat the victim for shock (pp.50–51) if necessary.

Support and reassure victim

Sitting position should help to ease victim's breathing

ANGINA PECTORIS

Meaning "a constriction of the chest," angina pectoris occurs when coronary arteries, which supply the heart muscle with blood, become narrowed and cannot carry a sufficient amount of blood to meet increased demands during exertion or excitement. An attack forces the victim to rest; the pain should ease soon afterward.

RECOGNITION

- Vicelike central chest pain, often spreading to the jaw and down one or both arms.
- Pain easing with rest.
- Shortness of breath.
- Weakness, often sudden and extreme.
- Feeling of anxiety.

+ YOUR AIMS

- To ease strain on the heart by ensuring that the victim rests.
- To obtain medical help if necessary.
- To help the victim with any medication.

⓪ WARNING

If the pain persists, or returns, suspect a heart attack (p.54).

DIAL 9·1·1 OR CALL EMS

Treat by giving the victim a full-dose (325 mg) aspirin tablet to chew. Constantly monitor and record vital signs – level of response, pulse, and breathing (pp.8–9).

If the victim becomes unconscious, open her airway and check breathing; be prepared to give rescue breaths and chest compressions if necessary (see LIFE-SAVING PROCEDURES, pp.19–48).

1 Help the victim sit down. Make sure she is comfortable and reassure her. This should help her breathing.

2 If the victim has medication for angina, such as tablets or a pump-action or aerosol spray, let her administer it herself. If necessary, help her take it.

Supervise and support victim as she takes medication

3 Encourage the victim to rest, and keep any bystanders away. The attack should ease within a few minutes.

ACUTE HEART FAILURE

In heart failure, the heart muscle is over-strained or damaged and cannot pump a sufficient amount of blood to the body. Fluid may build up in the lungs, making breathing difficult. A possible cause is a clot in a coronary artery (coronary thrombosis). Heart failure can occur suddenly.

RECOGNITION

- Severe breathlessness.
- Often, but not always, signs and symptoms of heart attack (p.54).

▶ Treat as for HEART ATTACK p.54

HEART ATTACK

A heart attack, known medically as a myocardial infarction, is most commonly caused by a sudden obstruction of the blood supply to part of the heart muscle. The main risk is that the heart will either stop beating or will be severely damaged.

The effects of a heart attack depend largely on how much of the heart muscle is affected; many victims recover completely if they are treated quickly in the hospital.

▶ See also LIFE-SAVING PROCEDURES pp.19–48

See also LIFE-SAVING PROCEDURES pp.19–48

RECOGNITION

- Persistent, vicelike central chest pain, often spreading to the jaw and down one or both arms. Unlike angina pectoris (p.53), the pain does not ease if the victim rests.
- Breathlessness and discomfort occurring high in the abdomen, which may feel similar to severe indigestion.
- Collapse, often without any warning.
- Sudden faintness or dizziness.
- A sense of impending doom.
- "Ashen" skin, and blueness at the lips.
- A rapid, weak, or irregular pulse.
- Profuse sweating.
- Extreme gasping for air.

+ YOUR AIMS

- To encourage the victim to rest.
- To arrange urgent transportation of the victim to the hospital.

ⓘ WARNING

If the victim becomes unconscious, open his airway and check breathing; be prepared to give rescue breaths and chest compressions if needed (see LIFE-SAVING PROCEDURES, pp.19–48).

Support victim with items such as pillows

1 Make the victim as comfortable as possible to ease the strain on his heart. A half-sitting position, with head and shoulders well supported and knees bent, is often best.

2 DIAL 9·1·1 OR CALL EMS State that you suspect a heart attack. If the victim asks you to do so, call his own doctor as well.

3 If the victim is fully conscious, give him a full-dose (325 mg) aspirin tablet and advise him to chew it slowly.

4 If the victim has medicine for angina, such as tablets or a pump-action or aerosol spray, help him take it. Encourage the victim to rest.

5 Constantly monitor and record vital signs – level of response, pulse, and breathing (pp.8–9) – until help arrives.

FAINTING

A faint is a brief loss of consciousness caused by a temporary reduction of the blood flow to the brain. Fainting may be a reaction to pain, exhaustion, lack of food, or emotional stress. It is also common after long periods of inactivity, such as standing or sitting still, especially in a warm atmosphere – blood pools in the legs, reducing the amount that reaches the brain.

When a person faints, the pulse rate becomes very slow. However, the rate soon picks up and returns to normal. A victim who has fainted usually makes a rapid and complete recovery.

▶ See also LIFE-SAVING PROCEDURES pp.19–48

RECOGNITION
- A brief loss of consciousness that causes the victim to fall to the floor.
- A slow pulse.
- Pale, cold skin and sweating.

＋ YOUR AIMS
- To improve blood flow to the brain.
- To reassure the victim as she recovers and make her comfortable.

1 When a victim feels faint, advise her to lie down. Kneel down, raise her legs, and support her ankles on your shoulders; this helps improve the blood flow to the brain.

Support ankles on your shoulders

Raise legs to improve blood flow to brain

Watch face for signs of recovery

2 Make sure that the victim has plenty of fresh air; ask someone to open a window. In addition, ask any bystanders to stand clear.

3 As she recovers, reassure her and help her sit up gradually. If she starts to feel faint again, advise her to lie down again, and raise and support her legs until she recovers fully.

❶ WARNING
If the victim does not regain consciousness quickly, open her airway and check breathing; be prepared to give rescue breaths and chest compressions if necessary (see LIFE-SAVING PROCEDURES, pp.19–48).
DIAL 9-1-1 OR CALL EMS

ASTHMA

In an asthma attack, the muscles of the air passages in the lungs go into spasm and the linings of the airways swell. The airways become narrowed, making breathing difficult.

Victims usually treat their own asthma attacks, using a reliever inhaler. Preventer inhalers are used by victims to help prevent attacks; however, they are not an effective treatment for asthma attacks.

A diffuser or spacer can be fitted to the inhaler to help administer the medication.

✛ YOUR AIMS

• To ease breathing.
• To obtain medical help if necessary.

1 Keep calm and reassure the victim. Get her to take a puff of her reliever inhaler. It should relieve the asthma attack within a few minutes. Ask her to breathe slowly and deeply.

Use a spacer with the inhaler

Inhaler

2 Let her adopt the position that she finds most comfortable – often sitting down. Do not make the victim lie down.

3 A mild asthma attack should ease within 3 minutes. If it does not, ask the victim to take another dose from the same inhaler.

❶ CAUTION

If this is the first attack, or if the attack is severe and any one of the following occurs:

• the inhaler has no effect after 5 minutes;
• the victim is getting worse;
• breathlessness makes talking difficult;
• she is becoming exhausted;

DIAL 9·1·1 OR CALL EMS

Help her use her inhaler every 5–10 minutes. Monitor and record her breathing and pulse every 10 minutes (pp.8–9).

❶ WARNING

If the victim loses consciousness, open her airway and check breathing; be prepared to give rescue breaths and chest compressions if necessary (see LIFE-SAVING PROCEDURES, pp.19–48).

DIAL 9·1·1 OR CALL EMS

If the victim is breathing, place her in the recovery position (pp.30–31). Monitor her vital signs – level of response, pulse, and breathing (pp.8–9) – until help arrives.

DROWNING

Death by drowning occurs when air cannot get into the lungs, usually because of a small amount of water. This may also cause spasms of the throat.

Water may gush from a rescued victim's stomach out through the mouth. This should be left to drain of its own accord. Do not attempt to force it from the stomach because the victim may vomit and then inhale it.

A victim should always receive medical attention even if he seems to have recovered at the time. Water in the lungs causes them to become irritated, and the air passages may begin to swell several hours later.

Victims may also need treatment for hypothermia (pp.108–110).

▶ See also HYPOTHERMIA pp.108–110
● LIFE-SAVING PROCEDURES pp.19–48

✛ YOUR AIMS

- To restore adequate breathing.
- To keep the victim warm.
- To arrange urgent removal to the hospital.

1 If you are rescuing the victim from the water to safety, keep her head lower than the rest of her body to reduce the risk of her inhaling water.

2 Lay the victim down on her back on a rug or coat. Open her airway and check breathing; be prepared to give rescue breaths and chest compressions if necessary (*see* LIFE-SAVING PROCEDURES, pp.19–48). If the victim is breathing, place her in the recovery position (pp.30–31).

3 Treat the victim for hypothermia; remove wet clothing if possible and cover her with dry blankets.

Position victim's head low and to one side so that water drains from her mouth

4 DIAL 9·1·1 OR CALL EMS even if she appears to recover fully.

Listen and feel for breathing

❶ WARNING

Water in the lungs and the effects of cold can increase resistance to rescue breaths and chest compressions: you may have to do both at a slower rate than normal.

PENETRATING CHEST WOUND

The heart and lungs, and the major blood vessels around them, lie within the chest (thorax), protected by the breastbone and the ribcage, which extends downward to protect organs in the upper abdomen such as the liver and spleen. Penetrating wounds can cause severe internal damage. The lungs are particularly susceptible and damage to them causes breathing difficulties; it may also impair the operation of the heart, causing shock.

▶ See also LIFE-SAVING PROCEDURES pp.19–48 ● SHOCK pp.50–51

RECOGNITION

● Difficult and painful breathing, possibly rapid, shallow, and uneven.
● Victim feels an acute sense of alarm.
● Features of hypoxia, including gray–blue skin coloration (cyanosis).
There may also be:
● Coughed-up frothy, red blood.
● A crackling feeling of the skin around the site of the wound, caused by air collecting in the tissues.
● Blood bubbling out of the wound.
● Sound of air being sucked into the chest as the victim inhales.
● Veins in the neck becoming prominent.

✚ YOUR AIMS

● To seal the wound and maintain breathing.
● To minimize shock.
● To arrange urgent removal to the hospital.

❶ WARNING

If the victim becomes unconscious, open his airway and check breathing; be prepared to give rescue breaths and chest compressions, if necessary (*see* LIFE-SAVING PROCEDURES, pp.19–48). If he is breathing, place him in the recovery position (pp.30–31) on his injured side to help the healthy lung work effectively.

1 Put on disposable gloves if available. Lean the victim toward the injured side and cover the wound with his palm.

Completely cover the wound to prevent air from being drawn into the chest cavity

2 Place a sterile dressing or nonfluffy clean pad over the wound and surrounding area. Cover with a plastic bag, foil, or a sheet. Secure firmly with adhesive tape on three edges.

Leave fourth side untaped to allow air under pressure during exhaling to escape

3 DIAL 9·1·1 OR CALL EMS While waiting for help, continue to support the victim in the same position as long as he remains conscious.

4 Monitor and record vital signs – level of response, pulse, and breathing (pp.8–9) – until medical help arrives.

4

B REAKS IN THE SKIN or inner body surfaces are known as wounds. Open wounds allow blood and other fluids to be lost from the body and enable germs to enter. In a closed wound, bleeding is confined within the body tissues and is most easily recognized by bruising. Wounds can be daunting, particularly if there is a lot of bleeding, but prompt action will reduce blood loss and minimize shock.

UNDERSTANDING TREATMENT
The way in which injury is inflicted and the force exerted determine the effect of the wound on the body and how to treat it. Treatments for all types of wound are covered in this chapter. Always follow good hygiene procedures to guard against infection: wash your hands and wear disposable gloves if available.

CONTENTS

WOUNDS AND BLEEDING

> ### FIRST-AID PRIORITIES
>
> • Assess the victim's condition.
> • Comfort and reassure the victim.
> • Be careful about hygiene; wear gloves.
> • Control blood loss by applying pressure and elevating the injured part.
> • Minimize shock.
> • Obtain medical help, if necessary. Dial 9·1·1 or call your local EMS if you suspect a serious illness or injury.

SEVERE BLEEDING

When bleeding is severe, it can be dramatic and distressing. Shock is likely to develop, and the victim may lose consciousness. If bleeding is not controlled, the victim's heart could stop. Bleeding at the face or neck may impede the air flow to the lungs.

When treating severe bleeding, always check first whether there is an object embedded in the wound; take care not to press on the object.

▶ See also LIFE-SAVING PROCEDURES pp.19–48 ● SHOCK pp.50–51

IF NO OBJECT IS EMBEDDED IN WOUND

✚ YOUR AIMS

- To control bleeding.
- To prevent/minimize the effects of shock.
- To minimize infection.
- To arrange transportation to the hospital.

1 Put on disposable gloves if available. Remove or cut clothing as necessary to expose the wound.

2 Apply direct pressure over the wound with your fingers or palm, preferably over a sterile dressing or nonfluffy, clean pad (but do not waste any time looking for a dressing). You can ask the victim to apply direct pressure herself.

3 Raise and support the injured limb above the level of the victim's heart to reduce blood loss. Handle the limb very gently if you suspect that there is a fracture.

4 Help the victim lie down on a blanket, if available, to protect her from the cold. If you suspect that shock may develop, raise and support her legs so that they are above the level of her heart.

Keep injured limb raised

Maintain pressure on dressing

Keep injured part raised

Hold dressing firmly over wound

5 Secure the dressing with a bandage that is tight enough to maintain pressure, but not so tight that it impairs the circulation (p.14). If further bleeding occurs, apply a second dressing on top of the first.

If using a pad, cover it completely with bandage

6 If blood seeps through the second dressing, apply direct pressure again to the point of bleeding (see step 2, opposite).

7 Support the injured part and keep it raised with a sling and/or bandaging.

8 DIAL 9·1·1 OR CALL EMS Regularly monitor and record vital signs – level of response, pulse, and breathing (pp.8–9). Watch for signs of shock (pp.50–51), and check the dressings for seepage. Always check the circulation beyond the bandage (p.14).

> **! CAUTION**
>
> Do not give the victim anything to eat, drink, or smoke.

IF AN OBJECT IS EMBEDDED IN WOUND

> **+ YOUR AIMS**
>
> • To control bleeding without pressing the object into the wound.
> • To prevent/minimize the effects of shock.
> • To minimize infection.
> • To arrange transportation to the hospital.

1 Put on disposable gloves if available. Press firmly on either side of the object to push the edges of the wound together.

2 If the injury is to a victim's limb, raise and support the limb above the level of her heart to reduce the blood loss.

3 If possible, help the victim lie down on a blanket to protect her from the cold. If you suspect that shock may develop, raise and support her legs so that they are above the level of her heart.

4 Build up padding on either side of the object. Carefully bandage over the object without pressing on it.

Take care not to press on object

5 Support the injured part in a raised position with a sling and/or bandaging to help minimize swelling.

6 DIAL 9·1·1 OR CALL EMS Monitor and record vital signs – level of response, pulse, and breathing (pp.8–9). Watch for signs of shock (pp.50–51), and check the dressing for seepage. Check the circulation beyond the bandage (p.14).

CUTS AND SCRAPES

Bleeding from small cuts and scrapes is controlled by pressure and elevation. An adhesive dressing is normally all that is necessary, and the wound will heal in a few days. Medical aid need be sought only if:
- The bleeding does not stop.
- There is a foreign object embedded in the cut (opposite).
- The wound is at particular risk of infection (such as a human or animal bite, or a puncture by a dirty object).
- An old wound shows signs of becoming infected.

TETANUS

This is a dangerous infection caused by the bacterium *Clostridium tetani*. If tetanus bacteria enter a wound, they may multiply and release a poisonous substance (toxin) that spreads through the nervous system, causing muscle spasms and paralysis.

The disorder can be prevented by immunization, and people are normally given a course of tetanus immunization during childhood. However, immunization may need to be repeated in adulthood.

✛ YOUR AIM
- To minimize the risk of infection.

---

1 Wash your hands thoroughly, and put on disposable gloves if available.

2 If the wound is dirty, clean it by rinsing lightly under running water, or using an alcohol-free wipe. Then pat the wound dry using a gauze swab and cover with sterile gauze.

Rinse loose foreign particles away with water

---

❶ CAUTION

Always ask about tetanus immunization.
Seek medical advice if:
- The victim has never been immunized.
- The victim is uncertain about the timing and number of injections given.
- It is more than 10 years since the victim's last injection.

---

3 Elevate the injured part above the level of the heart, if possible. Avoid touching the wound directly. Support the affected limb with one hand.

Keep injured part raised

4 Clean the surrounding area with soap and water, wiping away from the wound. Pat dry. Remove the wound covering and apply an adhesive dressing. If there is a special risk of infection, advise the victim to see her doctor.

Wipe away from wound

Protect cleaned area with gauze before applying dressing

FOREIGN OBJECT IN A CUT

Always remove small foreign objects, such as small pieces of glass or grit, from wounds before giving treatment. If such items remain in a wound, they may cause infection or delayed healing in the short term and discoloration in the long term. Remove superficial pieces of glass or grit with tweezers. Alternatively, carefully pick the pieces off the wound or rinse them off with cold water. Do not remove objects that are firmly embedded in the wound because you may damage tissue and aggravate bleeding. Instead, apply dressings or bandages around them.

▶ See also EMBEDDED FISHHOOK p.113
● SPLINTER p.112

✚ YOUR AIMS

- To control bleeding without pressing the object into the wound.
- To minimize the risk of infection.
- To arrange transportation to the hospital.

1 Put on disposable gloves if available. Control any bleeding by applying pressure on either side of the object and raising the injured part above heart level.

2 Cover the wound with gauze to minimize the risk of infection.

Lightly drape gauze over wound

❗ CAUTION

Always ask about tetanus immunization. *Seek medical advice if:*
- The victim has never been immunized.
- The victim is uncertain about the timing and number of injections given.
- It is more than 10 years since the victim's last injection.

3 Build up padding around the object until you are able to bandage over it without pressing down. Carefully hold the padding in place until you have completed the bandaging.

Keep injured arm raised

Use rolled-up dressings for padding

4 Arrange to take or send the victim to the hospital if necessary.

SPECIAL CASE

LARGE OBJECTS
If the object is particularly large, and you cannot pad high enough to bandage over it without pressing on it, bandage around the object.

Avoid putting pressure on top of object

SCALP AND HEAD WOUNDS

The scalp has many small blood vessels close to the skin surface, so any cut can lead to profuse bleeding. This bleeding will often make a scalp wound appear worse than it is. However, in some cases, a scalp wound may form part of a more serious underlying injury, such as a skull fracture, or may be associated with a head or neck injury. For these reasons, you should examine a victim with a scalp wound very carefully, particularly if signs of a serious head injury may be masked by alcohol or drug intoxication. If you are in any doubt, follow the treatment for skull fracture (p.90). Also bear in mind the possibility of a neck (spinal) injury.

▶ See also SHOCK pp.50–51 • SKULL FRACTURE p.90 • SPINAL INJURY pp.79–81

✚ YOUR AIMS

- To control blood loss.
- To arrange transportation to the hospital.

❶ WARNING

If the victim becomes unconscious, open the airway and check breathing; be prepared to give rescue breaths and chest compressions if necessary (see LIFE-SAVING PROCEDURES, pp.19–48).

1 Put on disposable gloves if available. If there are any displaced flaps of skin at the injury site, carefully replace them over the wound. Reassure the victim.

Use pad larger than wound

Apply firm, steady pressure to bring bleeding under control

2 Cover the injury with a sterile wound dressing or a clean, nonfluffy pad. Apply firm, direct pressure on the pad. This measure will help control bleeding and reduce blood loss, minimizing the risk of shock developing.

3 Secure the dressing with a roller bandage. (For minor bleeding, you can keep the pad in place with a triangular bandage.)

Apply bandage that secures pad and maintains pressure

TRIANGULAR BANDAGE

4 Help the victim lie down, with his head and shoulders slightly raised. Take or send the victim to the hospital in the final treatment position. Regularly monitor and record the level of response, pulse, and breathing (pp.8–9).

EYE WOUND

The eye can be bruised or cut by direct blows or by sharp, chipped fragments of metal, stone, and glass.

All eye injuries are potentially serious because of the risk to the victim's vision. Even superficial abrasions on the eye's surface (cornea) can lead to scarring or infection. Do not touch or attempt to remove a foreign object that is embedded in the eye (p.114).

See also FOREIGN OBJECT IN THE EYE p.114

RECOGNITION

- Intense pain and spasm of the eyelids.
- Visible wound and/or bloodshot eye.
- Partial or total loss of vision.
- Leakage of blood or clear fluid from a wound.

YOUR AIMS

- To prevent further damage.
- To arrange transportation to the hospital.

1 Help the victim lie on her back, and hold her head to keep it as still as possible. Tell her to keep both eyes still; movement of the "good" eye will cause movement of the injured one, which may damage it further.

2 Ask the victim to hold a sterile wound dressing or clean, nonfluffy pad over the eye. If medical help will be delayed, secure the pad with a bandage but do not put pressure on the eye. Take or send her to the hospital in this position.

Use a large, soft pad that covers eye

BLEEDING FROM THE EAR

This usually occurs when an eardrum is burst (perforated), perhaps caused by a foreign object pushed in the ear, a blow to the side of the head, or an explosion. Symptoms include sharp pain, earache, deafness, and possibly dizziness. Watery blood is serious: it indicates that the skull is fractured and fluid is leaking from around the brain.

See also FOREIGN OBJECT IN THE EAR p.115 ● SKULL FRACTURE p.90

YOUR AIM

- To arrange transportation to the hospital.

① CAUTION

Do not tilt the victim's head if you suspect a skull fracture.

1 Help the victim into a half-sitting position, with his head tilted to the injured side so that blood drains away.

2 Put on gloves if available. Hold a sterile wound dressing or a clean, nonfluffy pad lightly in place on the ear. Send or take the victim to the hospital in the treatment position.

NOSEBLEED

Bleeding from the nose often occurs when blood vessels inside the nostrils rupture, perhaps as a result of sneezing or blowing the nose. Nosebleeds may also occur as a result of high blood pressure. A nosebleed can be dangerous if the victim loses a lot of blood.

If bleeding follows a head injury and the blood is thin and watery, this is serious: fluid leaking from around the brain indicates a fractured skull.

▶ See also FOREIGN OBJECT IN THE NOSE p.115

✚ YOUR AIMS

- To control blood loss.
- To maintain an open airway.

1 Ask the victim to sit down. Advise her to tilt her head forward to allow the blood to drain from the nostrils.

2 Ask the victim to breathe through her mouth (this will also have a calming effect) and to pinch the soft part of the nose. Reassure and help her if necessary.

Pinch just below hard part of nose

SPECIAL CASE

CHILDREN
A young child may be worried by a nosebleed. Try to reassure her and give her a bowl that she can spit or dribble into.

Pinch child's nose

3 Tell the victim to keep pinching her nose. Advise her not to speak, swallow, cough, spit, or sniff because she may disturb blood clots that have formed in the nose. Give her a clean cloth or tissue to mop up any dribbling.

4 After about 10 minutes, tell the victim to release the pressure. If the bleeding has not stopped, tell her to reapply the pressure for two further periods of 10 minutes each.

5 Once the bleeding has stopped, and with the victim still leaning forward, clean around her nose with lukewarm water.

6 Advise the victim to rest quietly for a few hours. Tell her to avoid exertion and, in particular, not to blow her nose, because these actions will disturb any clots.

❶ CAUTION

- Do not let the head tip back; blood may run down the throat and induce vomiting.
- If bleeding stops and then restarts, tell the victim to reapply pressure.
- If the nosebleed is severe, or if it lasts longer than 30 minutes in total, take or send the victim to the hospital in the treatment position.

ABDOMINAL WOUND

A knife, gunshot, or crush injury to the abdomen can puncture, lacerate or rupture organs and major blood vessels deep inside the body. The severity of a wound may be evident from symptoms such as external bleeding and protruding abdominal contents. More often, there is hidden internal injury and bleeding, which may be fatal if there is any delay in emergency treatment. There is also a high risk of shock and infection.

▶ See also SHOCK pp.50–51

✚ YOUR AIMS

- To minimize shock.
- To minimize the risk of infection.
- To arrange urgent removal to the hospital.

1 Put on disposable gloves if available. Help the victim lie down on a firm surface, preferably on a blanket. Loosen any tight clothing, such as a belt or a shirt.

Undo belt

Raise and support victim's knees to ease strain on injury

3 DIAL 9·1·1 OR CALL EMS Treat the victim for shock (pp.50–51). Regularly monitor and record vital signs – level of response, pulse, and breathing (pp.8–9).

2 Put a dressing over the wound, and secure it in place with a bandage or adhesive tape. If blood seeps through the dressing, apply another dressing or pad on top of the first one.

ⓘ WARNING

- If a victim with an open wound coughs or vomits, press on the dressing to prevent the contents of the abdomen from pushing through the wound and being exposed.

- Do not touch any intestine protruding from the abdomen. Cover the area with a clean plastic bag. Alternatively, apply a sterile wound dressing.

- If the victim becomes unconscious, open the airway and check breathing; be ready to give rescue breaths and chest compressions if needed (see LIFE-SAVING PROCEDURES, pp.19–48). If he is breathing, put him in the recovery position (pp.30–31), taking care to support the abdomen.

WOUND TO THE PALM

Because the palm has several large blood vessels, a wound here may cause profuse bleeding. There is also a risk that a deep wound to the palm may sever tendons and nerves in the hand and result in loss of feeling or movement in the fingers

▶ See also FOREIGN OBJECT IN A CUT p.63
● SHOCK pp.50–51

+ YOUR AIMS

- To control blood loss and minimize the effects of shock.
- To minimize the risk of infection.
- To arrange transportation to the hospital.

1 Put on disposable gloves if available. Press a sterile wound dressing or clean pad firmly into the palm, and ask the victim to clench his fist over it. If he cannot press hard, tell him to grasp his fist with his uninjured hand.

2 Bandage the victim's fingers so that they are clenched over the pad. Tie the ends of the bandage over the top of the fingers.

Leave thumb free

Raise and support arm

3 Support the victim's arm in an elevation sling (p.18) to keep it raised. Take or send the victim to the hospital.

WOUND AT A JOINT CREASE

Major blood vessels inside the elbows and knees will bleed copiously if severed. The steps below help control bleeding and shock but, because they also impede blood flow to the lower part of the limb, you must keep checking circulation to this area.

▶ See also FOREIGN OBJECT IN A CUT p.63
● SHOCK pp.50–51

+ YOUR AIMS

- To control blood loss and minimize the effects of shock.
- To minimize the risk of infection.
- To arrange transportation to the hospital.

1 Put on disposable gloves if available. Press a sterile wound dressing or clean pad on the injury. Bend the joint to hold the pad and keep pressure on the wound.

2 Raise and support the limb. If possible, help the victim lie down with his legs raised and supported.

3 Take or send the victim to the hospital in the final treatment position. Every 10 minutes, check the circulation beyond the injury. If needed, briefly release pressure on the wound to restore normal blood flow to the lower part of the limb, then reapply pressure.

5

THE SKELETON is the supporting framework around which the body is constructed. It is jointed in many places, and muscles attached to the bones enable us to move. Most of our movements are controlled at will and coordinated by impulses that travel from the brain via the nerves to every muscle and joint in the body.

DIAGNOSING TYPES OF INJURY
Because it is sometimes difficult to distinguish between bone, joint, and muscle injuries, the chapter begins with an overview of the types of injury. First-aid treatments for most injuries, from major fractures to sprains and dislocations, are given here. Skull fracture is covered in the chapter on disorders of consciousness (p.90) because of the potential damage to the brain that this injury can cause.

CONTENTS

BONE, JOINT, AND MUSCLE INJURIES

✚ FIRST-AID PRIORITIES

• Assess the victim's condition.
• Comfort and reassure the victim.
• Steady and support the injured part.
• Enhance the support with padding, bandages, and splints if necessary.
• Minimize shock.
• Obtain medical aid if necessary. Dial 9·1·1 or call EMS if you suspect a serious injury.

TYPES OF INJURY

A break or crack in a bone is known as a fracture. Bones are not brittle like chalk, but tough and resilient. When struck or twisted, they bend like branches. This means that generally, considerable force is needed to break a bone, unless it is diseased or old. Growing bones, however, are supple and may split, bend, or crack.

A joint may become dislocated, with the bones being partially or completely pulled out of position. Dislocation can result from the bone being wrenched into an abnormal position or violent muscle contraction.

Strains and sprains result from injury to, or overstretching of, the muscles, ligaments, or tendons.

FRACTURES

A bone may break at the point where a heavy blow is received – for example, when struck by a car (direct force). Fractures may also result from a twist or a wrench (indirect force).

STABLE AND UNSTABLE FRACTURES
In a stable fracture, the broken bone ends do not move because they are incompletely broken or jammed together. Usually, they can be gently treated without causing more damage.

In an unstable fracture, the broken bone ends can easily move out of position. As a result, there is a risk that they may damage blood vessels, nerves, and organs. Unstable injuries

can occur if the bone is completely broken or the ligaments are torn (ruptured). Handle these injuries very carefully to avoid further damage.

OPEN AND CLOSED FRACTURES
In an open fracture, one of the broken bone ends may pierce the skin surface, or there may be a wound at the fracture site, carrying a high risk of infection.

In a closed fracture, the skin above the fracture is intact. However, bones may be displaced (unstable) and damage internal tissues. If the bone ends pierce organs or major blood vessels, the victim may have internal bleeding and suffer shock (pp.50–51).

Pelvis   Hip joint   Thigh bone

Stable injury
Although the bone is fractured, the ends of the injury remain in place. The risk of bleeding or further damage is minimal.

Unstable injury
In this type of fracture, the broken bone ends can easily be displaced by movement or muscle contraction, which can lead to further damage.

Closed fracture
The skin is not broken, although the bone ends may damage nearby tissues and blood vessels. Internal bleeding is a risk.

Open fracture
Bone is exposed at the surface where it breaks the skin. The victim is likely to suffer bleeding. Infection is a risk.

DISLOCATIONS

These very painful injuries often affect the shoulder (*see* SHOULDER INJURY, p.74), jaw, hip, or joints in the thumbs or fingers. Dislocations may be associated with torn ligaments (see below) or damage to the synovial membrane, which lines the joint capsule. In some cases, joint dislocation can be serious. Dislocation of major joints may damage major nerves that supply the limbs and result in paralysis. A severe dislocation may also fracture the bones involved.

It can be difficult to distinguish a dislocation from a closed fracture. If in doubt, treat the injury as a fracture.

MUSCLE, TENDON, AND LIGAMENT INJURIES

The softer structures around bones and joints – the ligaments, muscles, and tendons – may be injured in several ways. Injuries to these soft tissues are commonly called strains and sprains (p.72). They occur when the tissues are overstretched and partially or completely torn (ruptured) by violent or sudden movements.

LIGAMENT INJURY

Ligaments connect bones at a joint. They may be torn in a sudden or unexpected wrenching that pulls the bones in the joint too far apart and tears the surrounding tissues.

Sprained ankle
This is due to overstretching or tearing of a ligament – the fibrous cords that connect bones at a joint. In this example, one of the ligaments in the ankle is partially torn.

MUSCLE AND TENDON INJURY
Muscles and tendons (which attach muscle to bone) may be bruised, strained, or ruptured. A strain often occurs at the point where the tendon attaches to the bone. In a rupture, a muscle or tendon is torn completely; this may occur in the main bulk of the muscle or in the tendon.

Ruptured extensor tendon

Finger joint

Phalanx

Torn finger tendon
Tendons attach muscle to bone across a joint. If a hard object strikes the end of the finger, the extensor tendon, which passes over the top of the finger joint, may be torn from its attachment.

Normal muscle fibers

Torn muscle fibers produce localized pain and swelling

Muscle tears
Vigorous movements may cause muscle fibers to tear. Muscle tears can cause severe pain and swelling.

Fibula

Sprained ligament

Heel bone

STRAINS AND SPRAINS

Ligaments, muscles, and tendons can be overstretched and partially or completely torn (ruptured) by violent or sudden movements. Deep bruising may be extensive in parts of the body where there is a large bulk of muscle. Such injuries are usually accompanied by bleeding into surrounding tissues, which can lead to pain, swelling, and bruising. Follow the "RICE" procedure to treat sprains and strains:

R – *Rest* the injured part.
I – Apply *Ice* or a cold compress.

C – *Compress* the injury.
E – *Elevate* the injured part.
If you are in any doubt as to the severity of the injury, arrange to take or send the victim to the hospital.

YOUR AIMS

- To reduce swelling and pain.
- To obtain medical aid if necessary.

1 Advise the victim to sit or lie down. Support the injured part in a comfortable position.

Use your knee to support injured leg

2 If the injury has just happened, cool the area by applying an ice pack or cold pad (p.12). This will help reduce swelling, bruising, and pain.

3 Apply gentle, even pressure (compression) to the injured part by surrounding the area with a thick layer of soft padding, such as cotton or plastic foam, and securing this layer of padding with a bandage. Check the circulation beyond the bandaging (p.14) every 10 minutes.

Apply bandage to compress injured part

Support foot

4 Raise (elevate) and support the injured part to reduce the flow of blood to the injury. This action will help minimize bruising in the area.

5 If the pain is severe, or the victim is unable to use the injured part, take or send her to the hospital. Otherwise, advise the victim to rest and to see her doctor if necessary.

CHEEKBONE & NOSE FRACTURES

Fractures of the cheekbone and nose are usually the result of deliberate blows to the face. Swollen facial tissues are likely to cause discomfort, and the air passages in the nose may become blocked, making breathing difficult. These injuries should always be examined at the hospital.

RECOGNITION

There may be:
- Pain, swelling, and bruising.
- A wound or bleeding from the nose or mouth.

▶ See also NOSEBLEED p.66

✚ YOUR AIMS

- To minimize pain and swelling.
- To transport or send the victim to the hospital.

❶ CAUTION

If there is straw-colored fluid leaking from the victim's nose, treat the victim as for a skull fracture (p.90).

1 Gently apply a cold compress (p.12) to the injured area to help reduce pain and limit potential swelling.

2 If the victim has a nosebleed, try to stop the bleeding (p.66). Arrange to take or send the victim to the hospital.

LOWER JAW INJURY

Jaw fractures are usually the result of direct force, such as a heavy blow to the chin. In some cases, a blow to one side of the jaw may cause a fracture on the other side. A fall onto the point of the chin can fracture the jaw on both sides. The lower jaw may also be dislocated by a blow to the face, or sometimes by yawning.

RECOGNITION

There may be:
- Difficulty speaking, swallowing, and moving the jaw.
- Pain and nausea when moving the jaw.
- Displaced or loose teeth and drooling.
- Swelling and bruising inside and outside the mouth.

✚ YOUR AIMS

- To protect the airway.
- To arrange transportation to the hospital.

❶ CAUTION

Do not bandage padding in case the victim vomits or has difficulty breathing.

1 If the victim is not seriously injured, help him sit with his head well forward to allow fluids to drain from his mouth. Encourage the victim to spit out loose teeth, and keep them to send to the hospital with him.

2 Give the victim a soft pad to hold firmly against his jaw in order to support it.

3 Take or send the victim to the hospital, keeping his jaw supported.

FRACTURED COLLAR BONE

It is rare for a collar bone to be broken by a direct blow. Usually, a fracture results from indirect force. The fracture may be due to impact at the shoulder, for example, from a fall onto an outstretched arm. These injuries often occur in young people as a result of sports activities. The broken ends of the collar bone may be displaced, causing swelling and bleeding in the surrounding tissues, and distortion of the shoulder.

RECOGNITION

There may be:
- Pain and tenderness, increased by movement.
- Swelling and deformity of the shoulder.
- Attempts by the victim to relax muscles and relieve pain; she may support the arm at the elbow, and incline the head to the injured side.

▶ See also FRACTURES p.70

✚ YOUR AIMS

- To immobilize the injured upper limb.
- To arrange transportation to the hospital.

1 Help the victim sit down. Lay the affected arm diagonally across her chest with her fingertips resting against the opposite shoulder. Ask her to support the elbow with her other hand.

3 Carefully place some soft padding, such as a small towel or folded clothing, between the arm and the body to make the victim more comfortable.

4 Secure the arm to the chest with a binder bandage (p.16) tied around the chest and over the sling.

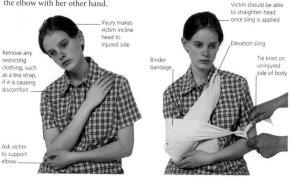

Injury makes victim incline head to injured side

Remove any restricting clothing, such as a bra strap, if it is causing discomfort

Ask victim to support elbow

Victim should be able to straighten head once sling is applied

Elevation sling

Binder bandage

Tie knot on uninjured side of body

2 Support the arm on the affected side in an elevation sling (p.18).

5 Arrange to take or send the victim to the hospital in a sitting position.

SHOULDER INJURY

A fall onto a shoulder or an outstretched arm, or a wrenching force, may pull the head of the arm bone (humerus) out of the joint socket. Ligaments around the shoulder joint may also be torn. This painful injury is called dislocation of the shoulder and requires hospital treatment.

A fall onto the point of the shoulder may damage the ligaments bracing the collar bone at the shoulder. Other shoulder injuries include damage to the joint capsule and to the tendons around the shoulder; these injuries tend to be common in older people and should be treated by following the RICE procedure (p.72).

⊳ See also SPRAINS AND STRAINS p.72

RECOGNITION

There may be:

- Severe pain, increased by movement, that may make the victim reluctant to move.
- Attempts by the victim to relieve pain by supporting the arm and inclining the head toward the injured side.
- A flat, angular look to the shoulder.

✚ YOUR AIMS

- To support the injured limb.
- To arrange urgent removal to the hospital.

❶ CAUTION

- Do not attempt to replace a dislocated bone into its socket.
- Do not allow the victim to eat, drink, or smoke because a general anesthetic may be necessary at the hospital.

1 Help the victim sit down. Gently place the arm on the affected side across her body in the position that is most comfortable.

2 Place a triangular bandage between the arm and the chest, in preparation for tying an arm sling (p.17).

3 Insert soft padding, such as a folded towel or clothing, between the arm and the chest, inside the bandage.

Sling is draped under the arm

Support arm while positioning padding

4 Finish tying the arm sling so that the arm and padding are well supported.

Site of injury

Keep bandage clear of injury site

5 Secure the limb to the chest by tying a binder bandage (p.16) around the chest and over the sling.

6 Arrange to take or send the victim to the hospital in a sitting position.

ARM INJURY

The most serious form of upper arm injury is a fracture of the long bone in the upper arm (humerus). It is common, especially in elderly people, for the arm bone to break at the shoulder end, usually in a fall.

The bones of the forearm (radius and ulna) can be fractured by an impact such as a heavy blow or a fall onto an outstretched hand. Since the bones have little fleshy covering, the broken ends may pierce the skin, producing an open fracture (p.70).

See also ELBOW INJURY opposite

RECOGNITION

There may be:
- Pain, increased by movement.
- Tenderness and deformity over the site of a fracture.
- Swelling and bruising.

At the wrist, the most common form of fracture is a Colles' fracture, which is a break at the end of the radius. In a young adult, a fall may break one of the small wrist bones (carpals).

YOUR AIMS

- To immobilize the arm.
- To arrange transportation to the hospital.

1 Ask the victim to sit down. Steady and support the forearm by placing it across his body. Expose and treat any wound that you find, wearing disposable gloves if available.

2 Place a triangular bandage between the chest and the injured arm, as for an arm sling (p.17). Surround the forearm in soft padding, such as a small towel or a thick layer of cotton.

Cradle arm in folds of soft padding

Ask victim to support injured arm

3 Fasten the sling around the arm and its padding using a square knot (p.16). Tie the knot at the hollow of the victim's collar bone on the injured side.

4 If the trip to the hospital is likely to be prolonged, secure the arm to the body by tying a binder bandage (p.16) over the sling, positioning it close to the elbow. Then take or send the victim to the hospital.

Tie binder bandage in front on uninjured side

ELBOW INJURY

A fracture or dislocation at the elbow usually results from a fall onto the hand. This is an unstable fracture (p.70), and the bone ends may damage blood vessels. Circulation in the arm must be checked regularly. In any elbow injury, the elbow will be stiff and difficult to straighten. Never try to force it to bend.

● See also ARM INJURY opposite

RECOGNITION

There may be

- Pain, increased by movement.
- Tenderness over the site of the fracture.
- Swelling, bruising, and deformity.
- Fixed elbow.

FOR AN ELBOW THAT CAN BEND

✚ YOUR AIMS

- To immobilize the arm without further injury to the joint.
- To arrange transport to the hospital.

● Treat as for ARM INJURY opposite

❶ CAUTION

Check the pulse in the affected wrist regularly (p.8). If the pulse is not present, gently straighten the elbow until the pulse returns. Support the arm in this position.

FOR AN ELBOW THAT CANNOT BEND

✚ YOUR AIMS

- To immobilize the arm without further injury to the joint.
- To arrange transportation to the hospital.

❶ WARNING

- Do not try to move the injured arm.
- Do not attempt to apply bandages if help is on its way.

1 Help the victim lie down. Place padding, such as towels, around the elbow for comfort and support.

Leave injury site free of padding

2 DIAL 9·1·1 OR CALL EMS
Check the pulse (p.8) in the injured arm until medical help arrives.

SPECIAL CASE

PREPARING FOR TRANSPORT
Put padding between the injured limb and body. Then use three folded triangular bandages to immobilize the injured limb against the trunk, at the wrist and hips (1), then above (2) and below (3) the elbow.

Tie bandages firmly on the noninjured side

HAND AND FINGER INJURIES

Minor fractures of the bones or joints in the hand are usually caused by direct force. The most common type – a fracture of the knuckle between the little finger and the hand – often results from a misdirected punch.

Multiple fractures are usually caused by crushing injuries. The fractures may be open, with severe bleeding and swelling, needing immediate first-aid treatment.

The joints in the fingers or thumb are sometimes dislocated or sprained as a result of a fall onto the hand.

RECOGNITION

There may be:
- Pain, increased by movement.
- Swelling, bruising, and deformity.
- In an open fracture, a wound and bleeding.

Always compare a suspected fractured hand with the normal hand because finger fractures result in deformities that may not be immediately obvious.

▶ See also DISLOCATED JOINT p.71
● FRACTURES p.70 ● WOUND TO THE PALM p.68

+ YOUR AIMS

- To immobilize and elevate the hand.
- To arrange transportation to the hospital.

1 If there is any bleeding, put on disposable gloves, if available. Apply a clean, nonfluffy dressing to the wound.

2 Remove any rings before the hand begins to swell, and then keep the hand raised to reduce swelling. Protect the injured area by wrapping the hand in folds of soft padding.

3 Gently support the affected arm across the victim's body by applying an elevation sling (p.18).

4 If necessary, secure the arm to the victim's body by tying a broad-fold bandage (p.16) around the chest and over the sling. Then arrange to take or send the victim to the hospital.

Use cotton or soft fabric as padding

Support wrist while treating hand

Ask victim to support injured arm by holding the elbow

Elevation sling

Keep binder bandage free of injury site and padding

SPINAL INJURY

Injuries to the spine can involve one or more parts of the neck and/or back: the bones (vertebrae), the disks of tissue that separate the vertebrae, the surrounding muscles and ligaments, or the spinal cord and the nerves that branch off from it.

The most serious risk associated with spinal injury is damage to the spinal cord. Such damage can cause paralysis and numbness below the injured area. The spinal cord or nerve roots can suffer temporary damage if they are pinched by displaced or dislocated disks or by fragments of broken bone. If the cord is partly or completely severed, the damage may be permanent.

WHEN TO SUSPECT SPINAL INJURY
The most important indicator is the mechanism of the injury. Always suspect spinal injury if abnormal forces have been exerted on the neck or back, and particularly if the victim

RECOGNITION

When the vertebrae are damaged, there may be:
● Pain in the neck or back at the injury site; this may be masked by other, more painful injuries.
● A step, irregularity, or twist in the normal curve of the spine.
● Tenderness in the skin over the spine.
When the spinal cord is damaged, there may be:
● Loss of control over limbs; movement may be weak or absent.
● Loss of sensation, or abnormal sensations such as burning or tingling. The victim may say that limbs feel stiff, heavy, or clumsy.
● Loss of bladder and/or bowel control.
● Breathing difficulties.

complains of any interference with feeling or movement. Take care to avoid unnecessary movement of the head and neck at all times.

SOME CAUSES OF SPINAL INJURY
Any of the following circumstances should alert you to the possibility of a spinal injury:
● Falling from a height.
● Falling awkwardly while doing gymnastics or using a trampoline.
● Diving into a shallow pool and hitting the bottom.
● Being thrown from a horse or motorbike.
● Being in a football tackle.
● Sudden deceleration in a vehicle.
● A heavy object falling across the back.
● Injury to the head or the face.

Structure of the spine
The spinal cord is protected by the vertebrae (back bones). Injury to a vertebra or to an intervertebral disk may damage nerve roots that emerge from the spinal cord or damage the cord itself.

Intervertebral disk
Spinal cord
Nerve root
Vertebra

Continued on next page

79

SPINAL INJURY (continued)

FOR A CONSCIOUS VICTIM

✚ YOUR AIMS

- To prevent further injury.
- To arrange urgent removal to the hospital.

❶ CAUTION

- Do not move the victim from the position in which you found her unless she is in danger.
- If the victim has to be moved, use the log-roll technique (opposite). Alternatively, use an orthopedic stretcher or backboard.

1 Reassure the victim and advise her not to move.
DIAL 9·1·1 OR CALL EMS

2 Kneel above the victim's head. Grasp the sides of the victim's head firmly, with your hands over the ears. Do not completely cover her ears – she should still be able to hear you. Steady and support her head in the neutral head position, in which the head, neck, and spine are aligned. This is the least harmful head position for a victim with a suspected spinal injury.

❶ WARNING

If you suspect neck injury, ask a helper to place rolled-up blankets, towels, or items of clothing on either side of the victim's head and neck, while you keep her head in the neutral position.

Continue to support the victim's head and neck until emergency medical technicians take over.

Support head throughout | Place rolled-up items against head and neck

3 Continue to support the victim's head in the neutral position until emergency medical technicians take over, no matter how long this may be. Get help to monitor and record her vital signs – level of response, pulse, and breathing (pp.8–9).

Rest arms on legs to keep them steady

Hold victim's head straight to steady the neck, but do not completely cover her ears

FOR AN UNCONSCIOUS VICTIM

YOUR AIMS

- To maintain an open airway.
- To resuscitate the victim if necessary.
- To prevent further spinal damage.
- To arrange urgent removal to the hospital.

SPECIAL CASE

LOG-ROLL TECHNIQUE
This technique should be used if you have to turn a victim with a spinal injury. Ideally, you need five helpers but the move can be done with three. While you support the victim's head and neck, ask your helpers to straighten her limbs gently. Then, ensuring that everyone works together, direct your helpers to roll the victim. Keep the victim's head, trunk, and toes in a straight line at all times.

1 Kneel above the victim's head. Grasp the sides of her head firmly with your hands over the ears. Steady and support her head in the neutral head position, in which the head, neck, and spine are aligned.

2 If necessary, open the victim's airway using the jaw thrust method. Place your hands on each side of her face with your fingertips at the angles of the jaw. Gently lift her jaw to open the airway. Take care not to tilt the victim's neck.

Gently lift jaw to open airway

Support head continuously

Give plenty of support at spine

Hold hip, thigh, and calf to steady leg

Ask helpers to space themselves evenly along victim's body

3 Check the victim's breathing. If she is breathing, continue to support her head. Ask a helper to DIAL 9·1·1 OR CALL EMS

4 If the victim is not breathing, and there are no signs of circulation, give rescue breaths and chest compressions (pp.19–48). If you have to turn the victim, use the log-roll technique (right).

5 Monitor and record vital signs – level of response, pulse, and breathing (pp.8–9) – until medical help arrives.

FRACTURED PELVIS

Injuries to the pelvis are usually caused by a direct or indirect force, such as in a car crash or by crushing. For example, the impact of a car dashboard on a knee can force the head of the thigh bone through the hip socket.

A fracture of the pelvic bones may be complicated by injury to tissues and organs inside the pelvis, such as the bladder. In addition, internal bleeding may be severe because there are major organs and blood vessels in the pelvis. Shock often develops as a result, and it should be treated promptly.

See also SHOCK pp.50–51

RECOGNITION

There may be:
- Inability to walk or stand, although the legs appear uninjured.
- Pain and tenderness in the region of the hip, groin, or back, which increases with movement.
- Blood at the urinary outlet, especially in a male victim. The victim may not be able to urinate or may find urination painful.
- Signs of shock and internal bleeding.

YOUR AIMS
- To minimize the risk of shock.
- To arrange urgent removal to the hospital.

CAUTION
Do not bandage the victim's legs together if this causes any more pain. In such cases, surround the injured area with soft padding such as clothing or towels.

1 Help the victim lie down on his back. Keep his legs straight and flat or, if it is more comfortable, help him bend his knees slightly and support them with padding, such as a cushion or folded clothing.

2 Place padding between the bony points of the knees and the ankles. Immobilize the legs by bandaging them together with folded triangular bandages; secure the feet and ankles (1), then the knees (2).

3 DIAL 9·1·1 OR CALL EMS Treat the victim for shock (pp.50–51).

4 Monitor and record vital signs – level of response, breathing, and pulse (pp.8–9) – until help arrives.

Tie binder bandage at knees

Tie cravat bandage in figure-eight at feet

Place soft padding between knees

Keep head flat to minimize risk of shock

HIP AND THIGH INJURIES

The most serious injury of the thigh bone (femur) is a fracture. It takes a considerable force, such as a traffic incident or a fall from a height, to fracture the shaft of the femur. This is a serious injury because the broken bone ends can pierce major blood vessels, causing heavy blood loss, and shock (pp.50–51) may result.

In the hip joint, the most serious, though much less common, type of injury is dislocation.

● See also DISLOCATED JOINT p.71
● FRACTURES p.70 ● SHOCK pp.50–51

RECOGNITION

There may be:
● Pain at the site of the injury.
● Inability to walk.
● Signs of shock.
● Shortening of the leg and outward turning of the knee and foot, as powerful muscles move the broken bone ends over each other.

+ YOUR AIMS

● To immobilize the lower limb.
● To arrange urgent removal to the hospital.

❶ WARNING

● Do not allow the victim to eat, drink, or smoke because he may need to have a general anesthetic in the hospital.
● Do not raise the victim's legs, even if he shows any signs of shock, because you may cause further internal damage.

1 Help the victim lie down. If possible, ask a helper to gently steady and support the injured limb. Gently straighten his lower leg.

2 DIAL 9·1·1 OR CALL EMS
If the ambulance is expected to arrive quickly, support the leg in the same position until the ambulance arrives.

3 If the ambulance is not expected to arrive quickly, immobilize the leg by splinting it to the uninjured one. Gently bring the sound limb alongside the injured one. Position bandages at the ankles and feet (1), then the knees (2). Add bandages above (3) and below (4) the fracture site. Insert soft padding between the legs to prevent the bony parts from rubbing against each other, then tie the bandages on the uninjured side.

4 Treat the victim for shock (pp.50–51): insulate him from the cold with blankets or clothing, but do not raise his legs.

Tie feet together with cravat bandage in figure-eight

Knot bandage on uninjured side

Fracture site

Binder bandages

Place soft padding between legs

83

KNEE INJURY

The knee is the hinge joint between the thigh bone (femur) and shin bone (tibia). The knee is supported by strong muscles and ligaments and protected at the front by a disk of bone called the kneecap (patella). Disks of cartilage protect the surfaces of the major bones. These structures may be damaged by direct blows, violent twists, or sprains. Possible knee injuries include fracture of the bones, sprains, and damage to the cartilage.

The victim may be unable to bend an injured knee joint; you should

There may be:
- Pain, spreading from the injury to become deep-seated in the joint.
- If the bent knee has "locked," acute pain on attempting to straighten the leg.
- Rapid swelling at the knee joint.

ensure that the victim does not try to walk on the injured leg.

Bleeding or fluid in the knee joint may cause swelling around the knee.

▶ See also SPRAINS AND STRAINS p.72

YOUR AIMS
- To protect the knee in the most comfortable position.
- To arrange removal to the hospital.

⚠ WARNING
- Do not attempt to straighten the knee forcibly. Displaced cartilage or internal bleeding may make it impossible to straighten the knee joint safely.
- Do not allow the victim to eat, drink, or smoke because she may need a general anesthetic at the hospital.
- Do not allow the victim to walk.

1 Help the victim lie down, preferably on a blanket to insulate her from the ground. Place soft padding, such as a pillow, blanket, or coat, under her injured knee to support it in the most comfortable position.

2 Wrap padding around the joint, and secure it with bandages that extend from mid-thigh to the middle of the lower leg to splint the leg.

3 Arrange removal of the victim to the hospital. The victim needs to remain in the treatment position, so she should be transported in an ambulance.

Use roller bandage to hold padding in place

Support victim's knee with soft padding

LOWER LEG INJURY

Injuries to the lower leg include fractures of the shin bone (tibia) and the splint bone (fibula), and tearing of the soft tissues. Fractures of the tibia are usually due to a heavy blow and are likely to produce a wound. The fibula can be broken by the twisting that sprains an ankle.

YOUR AIMS

- To immobilize the leg.
- To arrange urgent removal to the hospital.

1 Help the victim lie down, and carefully steady and support the injured leg. If there is an open wound, gently expose the wound and treat bleeding. Apply padding to protect the injury.

Support leg at knee and ankle

2 DIAL 9·1·1 OR CALL EMS Support the injured leg with your hands to prevent any movement of the fracture site. Maintain this support until the ambulance arrives.

CAUTION

If the victim's journey to the hospital is likely to be long and rough, place soft padding on the inside of the injured leg, from the knee to the foot. Secure legs with binder bandages as described above.

3 If the ambulance is delayed, support the injured leg by splinting it to the other leg. Bring the uninjured limb alongside the injured one and slide bandages under both legs. Place bandages at the feet and ankles (1), then knees (2). Add bandages above (3) and below (4) the fracture. Insert padding between the lower legs. Then tie the bandages firmly, knotting them on the uninjured side.

Use folded towel or clothing as padding

Cravat bandage in figure-eight

Binder bandage

Keep bandages clear of fracture site

SPECIAL CASE

SUSPECTED FRACTURE NEAR ANKLE
Place separate bandages above the ankle and around the feet, rather than one figure-eight.

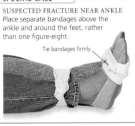

Tie bandages firmly

ANKLE INJURY

If the ankle is broken, treat it as a fracture of the lower leg (p.85). A more common injury is a sprain (p.72), which can be treated with the RICE procedure: *Rest* the affected part, apply *Ice*, *Compress* with bandaging, and *Elevate* (below).

RECOGNITION

- Pain, increased either by movement or by putting weight on the foot.
- Swelling.

See also SPRAINS AND STRAINS p.72

YOUR AIMS

- To relieve pain and swelling.
- To obtain medical aid if necessary.

CAUTION

If you suspect a broken bone, tell the victim not to put weight on the leg. Secure and support the lower leg (p.85), and take or send the victim to the hospital.

1 Rest, steady, and support the ankle in the most comfortable position.

2 If the injury has occurred recently, apply an ice pack or a cold compress (p.12) to the site to reduce swelling.

3 Wrap the ankle in thick padding and bandage firmly. Raise and support the limb. Advise the victim to rest the ankle and to see a doctor if pain persists.

FOOT AND TOE INJURIES

Fractures affecting the bones of the foot are usually caused by crushing. They are best treated at the hospital. When giving first aid, concentrate on relieving symptoms such as swelling.

RECOGNITION

- Difficulty walking.
- Stiffness of movement.
- Bruising and swelling.

YOUR AIMS

- To minimize swelling.
- To arrange transportation to the hospital.

1 Quickly raise and support the foot to minimize swelling.

2 Apply an ice pack or cold compress (p.12) to relieve swelling.

3 Arrange for the victim to go to the hospital. Ensure that the foot remains elevated during the trip.

Apply ice pack to reduce swelling

Use a soft item such as a cushion for comfortable support

Raise foot on firm items such as books

6

DISORDERS OF CONSCIOUSNESS

THE NERVOUS SYSTEM is the most complex system in the body. Its control center, the brain, is the source of consciousness, thought, speech, and memory. The brain also receives and interprets sensory information, which is carried by the nerves, and controls other body systems. If consciousness is impaired, even survival mechanisms, such as the cough reflex to keep the airway clear, may not function.

TREATMENT PRIORITIES

Because the problems described in this chapter can produce impaired consciousness, they need immediate attention. Your first-aid priorities are to monitor and maintain the vital functions of breathing and circulation and get medical help if necessary.

+ FIRST-AID PRIORITIES

- Assess the victim's condition.
- Comfort and reassure the victim.
- Maintain an open airway, check breathing, and be prepared to resuscitate if necessary.
- Protect the victim from harm.
- Look for and treat any injuries associated with the condition.
- Obtain medical aid if necessary. Dial 9·1·1 or call EMS if you suspect a serious illness or injury.

CONCUSSION

The brain moves a little within the skull and it can be "shaken" by a blow to the head, which is known as concussion. Common causes include traffic collisions, sports injuries, and falls. Concussion produces widespread temporary disturbance of normal brain activity but is usually not associated with any lasting damage to the brain. The victim will suffer impaired consciousness, but this usually lasts for only a few minutes and is followed by a full recovery.

A victim who has been concussed should be monitored and advised to obtain medical aid immediately should symptoms such as headache or blurred vision develop later.

See also CEREBRAL COMPRESSION pp.89
● LIFE-SAVING PROCEDURES pp.19–48
● SPINAL INJURY pp.79–81

RECOGNITION

● Brief period of impaired consciousness following a blow to the head.
There may also be:
● Dizziness or nausea on recovery.
● Loss of memory of events at the time of, or immediately preceding, the injury.
● Mild, generalized headache.

Mechanism of concussion
Concussion usually occurs as a result of a blow to the head. This "shakes" the brain within the skull, causing brain function to be disturbed temporarily.

YOUR AIMS

● To ensure the victim recovers safely.
● To place the victim in the care of a responsible person.
● To obtain medical aid if necessary.

WARNING

If the victim does not recover fully, OR if there is a deteriorating level of response after an initial recovery
DIAL 9-1-1 OR CALL EMS

CAUTION

All victims who have had a head injury should also be treated for a neck injury (see SPINAL INJURY, pp.79–81).

1 Perform a check of consciousness following the APVU code (p.8).

2 Monitor and record vital signs – level of response, pulse, and breathing (pp.8–9). Even if the victim appears to recover, watch him for subsequent deterioration in his level of response.

3 When the victim has recovered, place him in the care of a responsible person. If he has been injured playing sports, never allow him to continue without first obtaining medical advice.

4 Advise the victim to go to the hospital if he later develops symptoms such as headache, nausea, vomiting, or excessive sleepiness following a blow to the head.

CEREBRAL COMPRESSION

Compression of the brain, or cerebral compression, is very serious and almost invariably requires surgery. Cerebral compression occurs when there is a buildup of pressure on the brain. This pressure may be due to one of several different causes, such as an accumulation of blood within the skull or swelling of injured brain tissues.

Cerebral compression is usually caused by a head injury. However, it can also be due to other causes, such as a stroke (p.91), infection, or brain tumor. The condition may develop immediately after a head injury, or it may appear a few hours or even days later. For this reason, try to find out whether the victim has recently suffered a head injury.

▶ See also LIFE-SAVING PROCEDURES pp.19–48 ● SPINAL INJURY pp.79–81

Compression caused by bleeding
Bleeding may occur within the skull following a head injury or a disorder such as a stroke. The escaped blood may put pressure on brain tissues.

RECOGNITION

● Deteriorating level of response –
victim may become unconscious.
There may also be:
● History of a recent head injury.
● Intense headache.
● Noisy breathing, becoming slow.
● Slow, yet full and strong pulse.
● Unequal pupil size.
● Weakness and/or paralysis down one side of the face or body.
● High temperature; flushed face.
● Drowsiness.
● Change in personality or behavior, such as irritability or disorientation.

Accumulated blood may press on brain

Brain

Skull

✚ YOUR AIM

● To arrange transportation of the victim to the hospital.

❶ WARNING

If the victim is unconscious, open the airway using the jaw thrust method (p.81) and check breathing; be prepared to give rescue breaths and chest compressions (see LIFE-SAVING PROCEDURES, pp.19–48).
DIAL 9·1·1 OR CALL EMS
If breathing, try to maintain the airway in the position the victim was found.

1 DIAL 9·1·1 OR CALL EMS
If the victim is conscious, try to keep him supported in a comfortable resting position and reassure him.

2 Monitor and record the victim's vital signs – level of response, pulse, and breathing (pp.8–9) – regularly until medical help arrives.

❶ CAUTION

Do not allow the victim to eat, drink, or smoke because a general anesthetic may need to be given in the hospital.

SKULL FRACTURE

A skull fracture is very serious because there is a risk that the brain may be damaged either directly by fractured bone from the skull or by bleeding inside the skull. Clear fluid (cerebrospinal fluid) or watery blood leaking from the ear or nose are signs of serious injury.

You should suspect a skull fracture in any victim who has received a head injury resulting in impaired consciousness. Bear in mind that a victim with a possible skull fracture may also have a neck (spinal) injury and should be treated accordingly (*see* SPINAL INJURY, pp.79–81).

RECOGNITION

- Wound or bruise on the head.
- Soft area or depression on the scalp.
- Bruising or swelling behind one ear.
- Bruising around one or both eyes.
- Clear fluid (cerebrospinal fluid) or watery blood coming either from the nose or an ear
- Distortion or lack of symmetry of the head or face.
- Progressive deterioration in the level of response.

See also LIFE-SAVING PROCEDURES pp.19–48 • SCALP AND HEAD WOUNDS p.64 • SPINAL INJURY pp.79–81

YOUR AIMS

- To maintain an open airway.
- To arrange urgent removal of the victim to the hospital.

1 If the victim is conscious, help her lie down. Do not turn the head in case there is a neck injury.

2 Control any bleeding from the scalp by applying pressure around the wound. Look for and treat any other injuries. DIAL 9·1·1 OR CALL EMS

3 If there is discharge from an ear, cover the ear with a sterile dressing or clean pad, lightly secured with a bandage (*see* BLEEDING FROM THE EAR, p.65). Do not plug the ear.

4 Regularly monitor and record vital signs – level of response, pulse, and breathing (pp.8–9) – until medical help arrives.

WARNING

If the victim is unconscious, open the airway using the jaw thrust method (p.81) and check breathing; be ready to give rescue breaths and chest compressions if needed (*see* LIFE-SAVING PROCEDURES, pp.19–48).
DIAL 9·1·1 OR CALL EMS

Place your fingertips at the angles of the jaw

If the position in which the victim was found prevents maintenance of an open airway or you fail to open it using the jaw thrust, place her in the recovery position (pp.30–31). If you have helpers, use the "log-roll" technique (p.81).

STROKE

A "stroke" is a condition in which the blood supply to part of the brain is suddenly and seriously impaired by a blood clot or ruptured blood vessel. It is vital that the victim is taken to the hospital quickly. If the stroke is due to a clot, drugs may be given to limit the extent of the damage to the brain tissue and promote recovery.

Strokes are more common in later life and in people with circulatory disorders. The effect of a stroke depends on the extent of the damage to the brain. The condition can be fatal in some cases; however, many people make a complete recovery.

● See also LIFE-SAVING PROCEDURES pp.19–48.

RECOGNITION

There may be:
● Problems with speech and swallowing.
● If asked to show teeth, only one side of mouth will move or movement will be uneven.
● Loss of power or movement in the limbs.
● Sudden, severe headache.
● Confused, emotional mental state that could be mistaken for drunkenness.
● Sudden or gradual loss of consciousness.

✛ YOUR AIMS

● To maintain an open airway.
● To arrange urgent removal of the victim to the hospital.

❶ WARNING

If the victim is unconscious, open the airway and check breathing; be prepared to give rescue breaths and start chest compressions if needed (*see* LIFE-SAVING PROCEDURES, pp.19–48).

If she is breathing, place her in the recovery position (pp.30–31).

DIAL 9·1·1 OR CALL EMS

Monitor and record vital signs – level of response, pulse, and breathing (pp.8–9) – until medical help arrives.

❶ CAUTION

Do not give the victim anything to eat or drink because a stroke may make it difficult to swallow.

1 If the victim is conscious, help her lie down with her head and shoulders slightly raised and supported. Incline her head to the affected side, and place a towel on her shoulder to absorb any dribbling.
DIAL 9·1·1 OR CALL EMS

Victim may dribble on affected side

2 Loosen any clothing that might impair the victim's breathing. Continue to reassure her. Monitor and record vital signs – level of response, pulse, and breathing (pp.8–9) – until medical help arrives.

DIABETES MELLITUS

In this condition, the body fails to produce enough insulin, a chemical that regulates blood sugar (glucose) levels. As a result, sugar builds up in the blood, causing hyperglycemia (below). Too much insulin or too little sugar can cause hypoglycemia (opposite). The chart below compares both conditions. If a known diabetic victim appears unwell, give sugar. This will correct hypoglycemia and will do little harm in hyperglycemia.

COMPARING HYPERGLYCEMIA AND HYPOGLYCEMIA

Category		Hyperglycemia	Hypoglycemia
History	Recent eating habits	Eaten excessively	Undereaten or missed meals
	Amount of insulin used	Not enough for amount of food eaten	Too much for amount of food eaten
	Speed of onset of symptoms	Gradual	Rapid
Symptoms	Thirst	Present	Absent
	Hunger	Absent	Present
	Vomiting	Common	Uncommon
	Urination	Excessive	Normal
Signs	Odor on the breath	Fruity/sweet	Normal
	Breathing	Rapid	Normal
	Pulse	Rapid and weak	Rapid and strong
	Skin	Warm and dry	Pale and cold, with sweating
	Seizures	Uncommon	Common
	Level of consciousness	Drowsy	Rapid loss of consciousness

HYPERGLYCEMIA

High blood sugar (hyperglycemia) over a long period can result in unconsciousness. In most cases, the victim will drift into this state over a few days. Hyperglycemia requires urgent treatment in the hospital.

RECOGNITION

- Warm, dry skin; rapid pulse and breathing.
- Fruity/sweet breath and excessive thirst.
- If untreated, drowsiness, then unconsciousness.

✚ YOUR AIM

- To arrange urgent removal of the victim to the hospital.

1 DIAL 9·1·1 OR CALL EMS
If the victim is unconscious, place him in the recovery position (pp.30–31).

2 Monitor and record vital signs – level of response, pulse, and breathing (pp.8–9).

HYPOGLYCEMIA

When the blood-sugar level falls below normal (hypoglycemia), brain function is affected. This problem is characterized by a rapidly deteriorating level of response. Hypoglycemia can occur in people with diabetes mellitus and, more rarely, appear with an epileptic seizure or after an episode of binge drinking. It can also complicate heat exhaustion or hypothermia.

People with diabetes mellitus may carry their own blood-testing kits with which to check their blood-sugar levels, and many diabetics carry sugar lumps or a tube of glucose in gel form in case they feel they are having an attack.

If the hypoglycemic attack is at an advanced stage, consciousness may be impaired or lost and you must get emergency help immediately.

RECOGNITION

There may be.

- A history of diabetes; the victim may recognize the onset of a "hypo" attack.
- Weakness, faintness, or hunger.
- Palpitations and muscle tremors.
- Strange actions or behavior; the victim may seem confused or belligerent.
- Sweating and cold, clammy skin.
- Pulse may be rapid and strong.
- Deteriorating level of response.
- Diabetic's warning card, glucose gel, tablets, or an insulin syringe among victim's possessions.

▶ See also HEAT EXHAUSTION p.105 ● HYPOTHERMIA pp.108–110 ● LIFE-SAVING PROCEDURES pp.19–48 ● SEIZURES IN ADULTS pp.94–95

✚ YOUR AIMS

- To raise the sugar content of the blood as quickly as possible.
- To obtain medical aid if necessary.

❶ WARNING

- If consciousness is impaired, do not give the victim anything to eat or drink.
- If the victim is unconscious, open the airway and check breathing; be ready to give rescue breaths and chest compressions if necessary (see LIFE-SAVING PROCEDURES, pp.19–48). If she is breathing, place her in the recovery position.

DIAL 9·1·1 OR CALL EMS

Monitor and record the vital signs – level of response, pulse, and breathing (pp.8–9).

1 Help the victim sit or lie down. Give her a sugary drink, sugar lumps, chocolate, or other sweet food; or, if she has her own glucose gel, help her take it.

Give a sugary drink, which allows rapid absorption of sugar into blood

2 If the victim responds quickly, give more food or drink, and let her rest until she feels better. Advise her to see her doctor even if she feels fully recovered. If her condition does not improve, you should monitor her level of response (p.8) and look for other possible causes.

SEIZURES IN ADULTS

When many muscles in the body contract involuntarily, this is known as a seizure or a convulsion. The condition is due to a disturbance in the electrical activity of the brain. Seizures usually result in loss or impairment of consciousness. The most common cause is epilepsy. Other causes include head injury, some brain-damaging diseases, shortage of oxygen or glucose in the brain, and intake of certain poisons, including alcohol.

Epileptic seizures are due to recurrent, major disturbances of brain activity. Just before a seizure, a victim may have a brief warning period (aura) with, for example, a strange feeling or a smell or taste.

Care must include maintaining an open, clear airway and monitoring the victim's vital signs – level of response, pulse, and breathing. You will also need to protect the victim from further harm during a seizure and arrange care after he has recovered.

RECOGNITION

Generally:
- Sudden unconsciousness.
- Rigidity and arching of the back.
- Convulsive movements.

In epilepsy the sequence below is common:
- The victim suddenly falls unconscious, often letting out a cry.
- He becomes rigid, arching his back.
- Breathing may cease. The lips may show a gray–blue tinge (cyanosis) and the face and neck may become red and puffy.
- Convulsive movements begin. The jaw may be clenched, breathing may be noisy, and saliva – bloodstained if the mouth has been bitten – may appear. There may be loss of bladder or bowel control.
- Muscles relax, breathing becomes normal; the victim recovers consciousness, usually within minutes. He may feel dazed, act strangely, and be unaware of his actions.
- After a seizure, the victim may feel tired and fall into a deep sleep.

▶ See also LIFE-SAVING PROCEDURES pp.19–48

+ YOUR AIMS
- To protect the victim from injury.
- To give care when consciousness is regained.
- To get victim to the hospital if necessary.

1 If you see the victim falling, try to ease her fall. Make space around her and ask bystanders to move away. Remove potentially dangerous items, such as hot drinks and sharp objects. Note the time when the seizure started.

2 If possible, protect the victim's head by placing soft padding underneath it. Loosen clothing around her neck.

Loosen tight clothing around the neck

3 When the seizure has ceased, open the airway and check breathing; be ready to give rescue breaths and chest compressions if necessary (*see* LIFE-SAVING PROCEDURES, pp.19–48).

4 If she is breathing, place her in the recovery position. Monitor and record vital signs – level of response, pulse, and breathing (pp.8–9). Note the duration of the seizure.

> ⊘ **CAUTION**
>
> ● Do not move the victim unless she is in immediate danger.
> ● Do not put anything in her mouth or use force to restrain her.

> ⊘ **WARNING**
>
> *If any of the following apply*
> **DIAL 9-1-1 OR CALL EMS**
> ● The victim is unconscious for more than 10 minutes.
> ● The seizure continues for more than 5 minutes.
> ● The victim is having repeated seizures or having her first seizure.
> ● The victim is not aware of any reason for the seizure.

ABSENCE SEIZURES

Some people experience a mild form of epilepsy: seizures during which they seem unaware of their surroundings. These "absence seizures" tend to affect children more than adults. Convulsions or loss of consciousness are unlikely, but a full seizure may follow.

> **RECOGNITION**
>
> ● Sudden "switching off"; the victim may stare blankly ahead.
> ● Slight or localized twitching or jerking of the lips, eyelids, head, or limbs.
> ● Odd "automatic" movements, such as lip-smacking, chewing, or making noises.

> ✚ **YOUR AIM**
>
> ● To protect the victim from harm until she is fully recovered.

1 Help the victim sit down in a quiet place. Make space around her; remove any potentially dangerous items, such as hot drinks and sharp objects.

2 Talk to the victim in a calm and reassuring way. Stay with her until you are sure that she is fully recovered.

3 If the victim does not recognize or have any awareness of her condition, take her to the hospital.

SEIZURES IN CHILDREN

In young children, seizures – also called convulsions – are often the result of a raised body temperature associated with a throat or ear infection or other infectious disease. This type of seizure is known as a febrile convulsion and is a reaction of the brain to high body temperature. Epilepsy is another possible cause of seizures in infants and children.

Seizures can be alarming but they are rarely dangerous. However, the child should be seen at a hospital to rule out any serious underlying condition.

See also UNCONSCIOUS CHILD pp.32–39

RECOGNITION

- Violent muscle twitching, with clenched fists and an arched back.

There may also be:

- Obvious signs of fever: hot, flushed skin, and perhaps sweating.
- Twitching of the face with squinting, fixed, or upturned eyes.
- Breath-holding, with red, "puffy" face and neck or drooling at the mouth.
- Loss or impairment of consciousness.

➕ YOUR AIMS

- To protect the child from injury.
- To cool the child.
- To reassure the parents or caregiver.
- To arrange transportation to the hospital.

1 Position pillows or soft padding around the child so that even violent movement will not result in injury.

Use pillows or rolled blankets for padding

2 Remove any covering or clothes. Ensure a good supply of cool, fresh air (but do not overcool the child).

Undress him down to his briefs

3 Sponge the child's skin with tepid water to help cooling; start at his forehead and work down his body.

4 Once the seizures have stopped, keep the airway open by placing the child in the recovery position (pp.38–39) if necessary. **DIAL 9·1·1 OR CALL EMS**

5 Reassure the child and parents. Monitor and record vital signs – level of response, pulse, and breathing (pp.8–9) – until medical help arrives.

7

THIS CHAPTER DEALS with the effects of injuries and illnesses caused by environmental factors such as extremes of heat and cold.

The skin protects the body and helps maintain body temperature within a normal range. It can be damaged by fire, hot liquids, or caustic substances. Such injuries are often sustained in incidents such as explosions or chemical spillages.

The effects of temperature extremes can also impair skin and other body functions. The injuries may be localized – as in frostbite or sunburn – or generalized, as in heat exhaustion or hypothermia.

CONTENTS

ENVIRONMENTAL INJURIES

✚ FIRST-AID PRIORITIES

- Assess the victim's condition.
- Comfort and reassure the victim.
- Obtain medical aid if necessary. Dial 9·1·1 or call EMS if you suspect a serious illness or injury.

BURNS
- Protect yourself and the victim from danger.
- Assess the burn, prevent further damage, and relieve symptoms.

EXTREME TEMPERATURES
- Protect the victim from heat or cold.
- Restore normal body temperature.

SEVERE BURNS AND SCALDS

Take great care when treating burns that are deep or extensive. If the victim has been burned in a fire, assume that smoke or hot air has also affected the respiratory system (*see* BURNS TO THE AIRWAY, p.101).

The priorities are to begin rapid cooling of the burn and to check breathing. A victim with a severe burn or scald is likely to be suffering from shock and will need hospital care.

The possibility of nonaccidental injury must always be considered, no matter what the age of the victim.

Record all details accurately and retain any clothing that has been removed in case of future investigation.

▶ See also BURNS TO THE AIRWAY p.101
• LIFE-SAVING PROCEDURES pp.19–48
• SHOCK pp.50–51

✚ YOUR AIMS

• To stop the burning and relieve pain.
• To maintain an open airway.
• To treat associated injuries.
• To minimize the risk of infection.
• To arrange immediate removal to the hospital and to gather information for the emergency services.

ⓘ WARNING

Watch for signs of difficulty breathing; be prepared to give rescue breaths and chest compressions if necessary (*see* LIFE-SAVING PROCEDURES, pp.19–48).

1 Help the victim lie down. Try to prevent the burned area from coming into contact with the ground.

2 Douse the burn with cool water or other liquid for at least 10 minutes, but do not allow this to delay the victim's removal to the hospital. DIAL 9·1·1 OR CALL EMS

3 Continue cooling the affected area until the pain is relieved.

Use copious amounts of water to cool area and relieve pain

Place bowl under injured leg to catch water

Douse entire burned area repeatedly

4 Put on disposable gloves if available. Gently remove any rings, watches, belts, shoes, or smouldering clothing before the tissues begin to swell. Carefully remove any burned clothing, unless it is sticking to the burn.

Remove clothing around site of burn

Use blunt-tipped scissors to cut clothing

5 Cover the injured area with a sterile wound dressing to protect it from infection. If you do not have a sterile dressing, use a folded triangular bandage, part of a sheet, or a dressing; secure it with a bandage or adhesive tape applied over the dressing, not the skin.

> ### ❶ CAUTION
>
> • Do not over-cool the victim because you may lower the body temperature to a dangerous level. This is a particular hazard for babies and elderly people.
> • Do not remove anything sticking to the burn; you may cause further damage and introduce infection into the burned area.
> • Do not touch or otherwise interfere with the burned area.
> • Do not burst any blisters.
> • Do not apply lotions, ointment, butter, fat, or adhesive tape to the burned area.

> ### SPECIAL CASE
>
> BURNS TO THE FACE
> If the victim has a facial burn, do not cover the injury; you could cause the victim distress and obstruct the airway. Keep cooling the area with water to relieve the pain until help arrives.

Wear gloves to reduce risk of infection

Hold clean pad by edges to avoid infection

6 Gather and record details of the victim's injuries. Monitor and record her vital signs – level of response, pulse, and breathing (pp.8–9).

7 While waiting for help to arrive, reassure the victim and treat her for shock (pp.50–51) if necessary. Do not give her anything to eat.

MINOR BURNS AND SCALDS

Small, superficial burns and scalds are often due to domestic incidents, such as touching a hot iron or spilling boiling water on the skin. Most minor burns can be treated by first aid and will heal naturally. However, you should advise the victim to see a doctor if you are at all concerned about the severity of the injury.

Some time after a burn, blisters may form. These thin "bubbles" are caused

RECOGNITION

- Reddened skin.
- Pain in the area of the burn.

Later there may be:
- Blistering of the affected skin.

by tissue fluid (serum) leaking into the burned area just beneath the skin's surface. Do not break a blister: you may introduce infection into the wound.

YOUR AIMS

- To stop the burning.
- To relieve pain and swelling.
- To minimize the risk of infection.

❶ CAUTION

- Do not break blisters or otherwise interfere with the injured area.
- Do not apply adhesive dressings or adhesive tape to the skin; the burn may be more extensive than it first appears.
- Do not apply ointments, butter, or fats; they may damage tissues and increase the risk of infection.

1 Flood the injured part with cool water for at least 10 minutes to stop the burning and relieve the pain. This is more effective than using commercially prepared antiburn sprays.

2 Put on disposable gloves if available. Gently remove jewelry, watches, belts, or constricting clothing from the injured area before it begins to swell.

3 Cover the area with a sterile wound dressing or a clean, nonfluffy pad, and bandage loosely in place.

Gloves prevent cross infection through wound

Cover burn to keep out infection

Cool with plenty of water

SPECIAL CASE

BLISTERS
A blister usually needs no treatment. However, if the blister breaks or may burst, apply a nonadhesive dressing that extends well beyond the edges of the blister. Leave in place until the blister subsides.

BURNS TO THE AIRWAY

Burns to the face, and within the mouth or throat, are very serious because the air passages rapidly become swollen. Signs of burning will usually be evident. However, damage to the airway must be suspected if the victim has been burned in a confined space because he is likely to have inhaled hot air or gases.

For an extreme case, there is no specific first-aid treatment; swelling will rapidly block the airway, and there is a serious risk of suffocation. Immediate medical aid is required.

RECOGNITION

There may be:

- Soot around the nose or mouth.
- Singeing of the nasal hairs.
- Redness, swelling, or actual burning of the tongue.
- Damage to the skin around the mouth.
- Hoarseness of the voice.
- Breathing difficulties.

▶ See also LIFE-SAVING PROCEDURES pp.19–48 ● SHOCK pp.50–51

YOUR AIMS

- To maintain an open airway.
- To arrange urgent removal to the hospital.

⚠ WARNING

If the victim becomes unconscious, open the airway and check breathing; be prepared to give rescue breaths and chest compressions if necessary (*see* LIFE-SAVING PROCEDURES, pp.19–48). If the victim is breathing, place him in the recovery position (pp.30–31).

1 DIAL 9·1·1 OR CALL EMS
Tell the dispatcher that you suspect burns to the airway.

2 Take any steps possible to improve the victim's air supply, such as loosening clothing around his neck.

3 Reassure the victim. Monitor and record his vital signs – level of response, pulse, and breathing (pp.8–9) – until help arrives.

Reassure victim to keep him calm

Undo buttons at neck to ease breathing

ELECTRICAL BURN

Burns may occur when electricity passes through the body. While visible damage occurs at the points of entry and exit of the current, there may also be internal damage. The position and direction of entry and exit wounds may alert you to the likely site and extent of hidden injury and to the degree of shock the victim may suffer.

An electric shock can also cause cardiac arrest. If the victim is unconscious, your immediate priority, once you are sure the area is safe, is to open the victim's airway and check for breathing and circulation.

See also LIFE-SAVING PROCEDURES pp.19–48 • SEVERE BURNS AND SCALDS pp.98–99 • SHOCK pp.50–51

RECOGNITION

There may be:
- Unconsciousness.
- Full-thickness burns, with swelling, scorching, and charring, at the points of entry and exit.
- Signs of shock.
- A brown, coppery residue on the skin if the victim has been a victim of "arcing" high-voltage electricity. (Do not mistake this residue for injury.)

+ YOUR AIMS

- To treat the burns and shock.
- To arrange urgent removal to the hospital.

ⓘ WARNING

If the victim is unconscious, open the airway and check breathing; be prepared to give rescue breaths and chest compressions if necessary (see LIFE-SAVING PROCEDURES, pp.19–48).

1 Before touching the victim, first make sure that contact with the source of electricity is broken.

2 Flood the sites of injury, at the entry and exit points of the current, with cool water to cool the burns.

3 Put on disposable gloves if available. Place a sterile wound dressing, a clean, folded triangular bandage, or clean, nonfluffy material over the burns to protect them against airborne infection. DIAL 9·1·1 OR CALL EMS

4 Reassure the victim and treat him for shock (pp.50–51).

ⓘ CAUTION

Do not approach a victim of high-voltage electricity unless you are officially informed that the current is switched off and isolated.

Sweating may indicate shock

Cover burn with sterile dressing to protect from infection

Wash your hands or wear protective gloves

CHEMICAL BURN

Certain chemicals may irritate, burn, or penetrate the skin, causing widespread and sometimes fatal damage. Unlike burns caused by heat, signs of chemical burns may develop slowly, but the first aid is similar.

Most strong, corrosive chemicals are found in industry, but chemical burns can also occur in the home, especially from dishwasher products, oven cleaners, and paint thinner. Such burns are always serious and may

require urgent hospital treatment. If possible, note the name or brand of the burning substance. Always safeguard your own and others' health: some chemicals give off poisonous fumes.

RECOGNITION

There may be:
- Evidence of chemicals in the vicinity.
- Intense, stinging pain.
- Later, discoloration, blistering, peeling, and swelling of the affected area.

YOUR AIMS

- To make the area safe and inform the relevant authority.
- To disperse the harmful chemical.
- To arrange transportation to the hospital.

CAUTION

- Never attempt to neutralize acid or alkali burns.
- Do not delay the start of treatment by searching for an antidote.

4 Arrange to take or send the victim to the hospital. Make sure that the airway is open. Monitor vital signs – level of response, pulse, and breathing (pp.8–9). Pass on details of the chemical to medical staff. Call the Poison Control Center (800-222-1222) if you have any questions.

1 Make sure that the area around the victim is safe. Ventilate the area to disperse fumes, and, if possible, seal the chemical container. Remove the victim if necessary.

2 Flood the burn with water for at least 20 minutes to disperse the chemical and stop the burning. If treating a victim on the ground, ensure that the water does not collect underneath her.

3 Gently remove any contaminated clothing while flooding the injury.

Wear gloves to prevent chemicals from getting on your skin

Ask victim if she can identify chemical

Pour away from yourself to avoid splashes

CHEMICAL BURN TO THE EYE

Splashes of chemicals in the eye can cause serious injury if not treated quickly. They can damage the surface of the eye, resulting in scarring and even blindness.

The priority is to wash out (irrigate) the eye so that the chemical is diluted and dispersed. When irrigating the eye, put on protective gloves, if available, and avoid splashing contaminated rinsing water on you or the victim.

RECOGNITION

There may be:
- Intense pain in the eye.
- Inability to open the injured eye.
- Redness and swelling around the eye.
- Copious watering of the eye.
- Evidence of chemical substances or containers in the immediate area.

+ YOUR AIMS
- To disperse the harmful chemical.
- To arrange transportation to the hospital.

ⓘ CAUTION

Do not allow the victim to touch the injured eye or remove a contact lens.

1 Put on protective gloves if available. Hold the victim's affected eye under gently running cool water for at least 10 minutes. Take care to irrigate the eyelid thoroughly both inside and out. You may find it easier to pour the water over the eye using an eye irrigator or a glass.

2 If the eye is shut in a spasm of pain, gently but firmly pull the eyelids open. Be very careful that contaminated water does not splash the uninjured eye.

3 Ask the victim to hold a sterile eye dressing or a clean, nonfluffy pad over the injured eye. If it will be some time before the victim receives medical attention, bandage the pad loosely in position.

Secure dressing with bandage

Ensure that water drains away from face

4 Identify the chemical if possible. Then arrange to take or send the victim to the hospital.

HEAT EXHAUSTION

This disorder is caused by loss of salt and water from the body through excessive sweating. Heat exhaustion usually affects people who are not acclimatized to hot, humid conditions; people who are ill with vomiting or diarrhea are particularly susceptible.

A dangerous and common cause of heat exhaustion is the excessively high body temperature, and other physical changes, that result from taking drugs such as Ecstasy. In some cases, heat exhaustion can lead to heatstroke and may even cause death.

RECOGNITION

As the condition develops, there may be:
- Headache, dizziness, and confusion.
- Loss of appetite and nausea.
- Sweating, with pale, clammy skin.
- Cramps in the arms, legs, or the abdominal wall.
- Rapid, weakening pulse and breathing.

▶ See also HEATSTROKE p.106
● LIFE-SAVING PROCEDURES pp.19–48

✚ YOUR AIMS

- To replace lost body fluids and salt.
- To cool the victim if necessary.
- To obtain medical aid if necessary.

1 Help the victim to a cool place. Get him to lie down with raised legs.

2 Give him plenty of water; follow, if possible, with a weak salt solution (one teaspoon of salt per liter of water).

3 Even if the victim recovers quickly, ensure that he sees a doctor. If the victim's responses deteriorate, place him in the recovery position (pp.30–31). DIAL 9·1·1 OR CALL EMS

4 Monitor and record vital signs – level of response, pulse, and breathing (pp.8–9). Be prepared to give rescue breaths and chest compressions if necessary (*see* LIFE-SAVING PROCEDURES, pp.19–48).

Support victim's head as he drinks water

Raise his feet to improve blood flow to brain

Place cushion under his feet for comfort

105

HEATSTROKE

This condition is caused by a failure of the "thermostat" in the brain, which regulates body temperature. The body becomes seriously overheated, often due to high fever or exposure to heat. Heatstroke can also result from use of drugs such as Ecstasy. In some cases, heatstroke follows heat exhaustion when sweating ceases, and the body cannot be cooled by sweat evaporation.

Heatstroke can develop with little warning, causing unconsciousness within minutes of feeling unwell.

RECOGNITION

There may be:
- Headache, dizziness, and discomfort.
- Restlessness and confusion.
- Hot, flushed, and dry skin.
- Rapid deterioration in the level of response.
- Full, bounding pulse.
- Body temperature above 104°F (40°C).

▶ See also CHECKING TEMPERATURE p.9 ● DRUG POISONING p.119 ● LIFE-SAVING PROCEDURES pp.19–48

✚ YOUR AIMS

- To lower the victim's body temperature as quickly as possible.
- To arrange urgent removal to the hospital.

Continue to soak sheet

Make victim comfortable using cushions or pillows

1 Quickly move the victim to a cool place. Remove as much of his outer clothing as possible.
DIAL 9·1·1 OR CALL EMS

2 Wrap the victim in a cool, wet sheet and keep the sheet wet until his temperature falls to 100.4°F (38°C) under the tongue, or 99.5°F (37.5°C) under the armpit. If no sheet is available, fan the victim, or sponge him with cool water.

3 Once the victim's temperature appears to have returned to normal, replace the wet sheet with a dry one.

4 Monitor and record vital signs – level of response, pulse, and breathing (pp.8–9) – until help arrives. If his temperature rises again, repeat the cooling process.

❶ WARNING

If the victim becomes unconscious, open the airway and check breathing; be prepared to give rescue breaths and chest compressions if necessary (see LIFE-SAVING PROCEDURES, pp.19–48). If the victim is breathing, place him in the recovery position (pp.30–31).

FROSTBITE

With this condition, the tissues of the extremities – usually the fingers and toes – freeze due to low temperatures. In severe cases, this freezing can lead to permanent loss of sensation and gangrene (tissue death) as the blood vessels become permanently damaged.

Frostbite usually occurs in freezing or cold and windy conditions. People who are unable to move around are particularly susceptible. In many cases, frostbite is accompanied by hypothermia (pp.108–110).

RECOGNITION

There may be:
- At first, "pins-and-needles."
- Pallor, followed by numbness.
- Hardening and stiffening of the skin.
- A color change to the skin of the affected area: first white, then mottled and blue. On recovery, the skin may be red, hot, painful, and blistered. Where gangrene occurs, the tissue may become black due to loss of blood supply.

▶ See also HYPOTHERMIA pp.108–110

● YOUR AIMS

- To warm the affected area slowly to prevent further tissue damage.
- To arrange transportation to the hospital.

1 If possible, move the victim into warmth before you thaw the affected part. Do not place the part close to a source of direct heat.

2 Gently remove gloves, rings, and any other constrictions, such as boots. Warm the affected part with your hands, in your lap, or in the victim's armpits. Avoid rubbing the affected area because this can damage skin and other tissues.

Allow victim to warm affected part

3 Place the affected part in warm water at around 104°F (40°C). Dry carefully, and apply a light dressing of fluffed-up, dry gauze bandage.

Use water that is warm but not hot

4 Raise and support the affected limb to reduce swelling. An adult may take two acetaminophen pills for intense pain. Take or send the victim to the hospital.

● CAUTION

- Do not put the affected part near a source of direct heat.
- Do not attempt to thaw the affected part if there is danger of it refreezing.
- Do not allow the victim to smoke.

HYPOTHERMIA

This develops when the body temperature falls below 95°F (35°C). The effects vary depending on the speed of onset and the level to which the body temperature falls. Moderate hypothermia can usually be reversed. Severe hypothermia – when the core body temperature falls below 86°F (30°C) – can be fatal.

WHAT CAUSES HYPOTHERMIA
Hypothermia may develop over several days in poorly heated houses. Infants, homeless people, elderly people, and those who are thin and frail are particularly vulnerable. Lack of activity, chronic illness, and fatigue all increase the risk; alcohol and drugs can exacerbate the condition.

Hypothermia can be caused by prolonged exposure to cold out of doors, particularly when there is a high "windchill factor." Death from immersion in cold water may also be caused by hypothermia, not drowning.

▶ See also DROWNING p.57 • LIFE-SAVING PROCEDURES pp.19–48

TREATMENT WHEN INDOORS

✚ YOUR AIMS

• To prevent the victim losing any more body heat.
• To rewarm the victim slowly.
• To obtain medical aid if necessary.

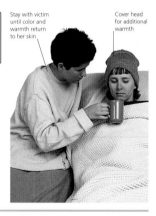

Stay with victim until color and warmth return to her skin

Cover head for additional warmth

1 For a victim who has been brought in from outside, quickly replace any wet clothing with warm, dry garments.

2 The victim can be rewarmed by bathing if she is young, fit, and able to climb into the bath unaided. The water should be warm but not too hot – about 104°F (40°C).

3 Put the victim to bed and cover her well. Give her warm drinks, soup, or high-energy foods to help rewarm her.

SPECIAL CASE

HYPOTHERMIA IN THE ELDERLY

An elderly person may develop hypothermia slowly over a number of days. Elderly people often have inadequate food or heating and are more likely to suffer from chronic illness that impairs their mobility.

When treating an elderly person with hypothermia, be careful to warm her slowly. Cover her with layers of blankets in a room at about 77°F (25°C). If the victim is warmed too rapidly, blood may be diverted suddenly from the heart and brain to the body surfaces.

Always call a doctor because hypothermia can sometimes disguise the symptoms of, or accompany, a stroke, a heart attack, or an underactive thyroid gland (hypothyroidism).

Warm an elderly victim gradually

❶ CAUTION

● Do not allow an elderly victim to have a bath to warm her up – the sudden warming may cause blood to divert suddenly from the heart and brain to the body surfaces.

● Do not place any heat sources, such as hot water bottles or fires, next to the victim because these may also mobilize blood too rapidly. In addition, they may burn the victim.

● Do not give the victim alcohol because this will worsen the hypothermia.

● Handle the victim gently because, in severe cases, rushed treatment or movement may cause the heart to stop.

4 Regularly monitor and record the victim's vital signs – level of response, pulse, breathing, and temperature (pp.8–9).

5 Call a doctor if you have any doubts about the victim's condition. If hypothermia occurs in an elderly person or a baby, you must always obtain medical aid for the victim.

SPECIAL CASE

HYPOTHERMIA IN INFANTS

Since a baby's mechanisms for regulating body temperature are underdeveloped, she may develop hypothermia in a cold room. The baby's skin may look healthy but feel cold, and she may be limp, unusually quiet, and refuse to feed. Rewarm a cold baby gradually, by wrapping her in blankets and warming the room. You should always call a doctor if you suspect a baby has hypothermia.

Cover head with a hat to prevent heat from being lost

Wrap the baby in a blanket

Continued on next page ⊙

ENVIRONMENTAL INJURIES

HYPOTHERMIA (continued)

TREATMENT WHEN OUTDOORS

✚ YOUR AIMS

- To prevent the victim from losing more body heat.
- To rewarm the victim.
- To obtain help.

❶ CAUTION

Do not give the victim any alcohol to drink. This is because alcohol dilates superficial blood vessels and allows heat to escape, making hypothermia worse.

❶ WARNING

If the victim becomes unconscious, open the airway and check breathing; be prepared to give rescue breaths and chest compressions if necessary (see LIFE-SAVING PROCEDURES, pp.19–48).

1 Take the victim to a sheltered place as quickly as possible.

2 Remove wet clothing. Shield the victim from the wind. Insulate him with extra clothing or blankets and cover his head. Do not give him your clothes.

3 Protect the victim from the ground and the elements. Put him in a dry sleeping bag, cover him with blankets or newspapers, and enclose him in a plastic or foil survival bag, if available.

Lay victim on a thick layer of dry insulating material, such as pine branches, heather, or bracken

Protect him from wind and rain with survival bag

Shelter and warm him with your body

4 Send for help. In an ideal situation, two people should go together for help. However, it is important that you do not leave the victim alone; someone must remain with him at all times.

5 To help rewarm a victim who is conscious, give him warm drinks, and feed him with high-energy foods, if you have appropriate drinks or foods available.

6 When help arrives, the victim should be taken to the hospital by stretcher immediately.

SPECIAL CASE

WHEN NO HELP IS AVAILABLE
If you are alone with the victim, try to attract attention by using a whistle, waving a flashlight, or lighting a fire.

8

CONTENTS

OBJECTS THAT FIND their way into the body, either through a wound in the skin or via an orifice (such as the ear, nose, or eye), are known as "foreign objects." Such items range from specks of dirt or grit in the eye to small objects that young children may push into their noses and ears. Foreign objects do not usually cause serious problems, but they can be painful and distressing. Calm, reassuring treatment is essential.

TREATMENT PROCEDURES
This chapter gives advice on how to remove objects from the skin and orifices, including what to do when something has been swallowed or inhaled. First aid for a person with an object embedded in a wound is given in Chapter 4, Wounds and Bleeding (pp.59–68).

＋ FIRST-AID PRIORITIES

- Assess the victim's condition.
- Comfort and reassure the victim.
- Establish whether or not a foreign object can be removed safely.
- Prevent further damage.
- Obtain medical aid if necessary. Dial 9·1·1 or call EMS if you suspect a serious illness or injury.

SPLINTER

Small splinters of wood, metal, or glass may enter the top layer of skin. They carry a risk of infection because they are rarely clean. Usually, a splinter can be withdrawn from the skin using sterile tweezers. However, if the splinter is deeply embedded in the skin, lies over a joint, or is difficult to remove, you should leave it in place and advise the victim to consult a doctor.

▶ See also FOREIGN OBJECT IN A CUT p.63

✛ YOUR AIMS

- To remove the splinter.
- To minimize the risk of infection.

1 Sterilize a pair of tweezers by holding them in a flame and then letting them cool. Put on disposable gloves if available. Gently clean around the splinter with soap and warm water.

Hold tweezers in flame

2 Grasp the splinter with the tweezers as close to the skin as possible, and draw it out at the angle at which it went in.

Pull out splinter in straight line, along the track of entry

Hold tweezers close to ends for better grip

SPECIAL CASE

EMBEDDED SPLINTER
If a splinter is embedded or difficult to dislodge, do not probe the area with a sharp object such as a needle or you may introduce infection. Pad around the splinter until you can bandage over it without pressing down, and seek medical advice.

3 Carefully squeeze the wound to encourage a little bleeding. This will help flush out any remaining dirt.

Encourage bleeding to flush out dirt

4 Clean the area, pat it dry, and apply an adhesive bandage to minimize the risk of infection.

❶ CAUTION

Always ask about tetanus immunization.
Seek medical advice if:
- The victim has never been immunized.
- The victim is uncertain about the timing and number of injections that have been given.
- It is more than 10 years since the victim's last injection.

EMBEDDED FISHHOOK

A fishhook is barbed, which means that once embedded in the skin it is difficult to remove. Only remove a hook yourself if medical aid is not available. Embedded fishhooks carry a risk of infection, including tetanus.

WHEN MEDICAL AID IS NOT READILY AVAILABLE

YOUR AIMS

• To remove the fishhook without causing the victim any further injury and pain.

WARNING

Do not try to pull out a fishhook unless you can cut off the barb. If you cannot, seek medical help.

1 Put on disposable gloves if available. If the barb is visible, use wirecutters to cut it away; carefully withdraw the hook by its eye.

Cut barb with wirecutters

Eye

2 Clean the wound, then pad around it with gauze and bandage it.

SPECIAL CASE

BARB NOT VISIBLE
Push the hook farther in until the barb emerges. Cut off the barb, and remove the hook (left). If you cannot do this, seek medical help.

Push quickly and firmly

CAUTION

Always ask about tetanus immunization. *Seek medical advice if:*
• The victim has never been immunized.
• The victim is uncertain about the timing and number of injections that have been given.
• It is more than 10 years since the victim's last injection.

WHEN MEDICAL AID IS READILY AVAILABLE

YOUR AIMS

• To obtain medical aid.
• To minimize the risk of infection.

1 Put on disposable gloves if available. Ask the victim to sit down and support the injured area. Cut off the fishing line, being careful to make the cut as close to the hook as possible.

2 Build up pads of gauze around the hook until you can bandage over it without pushing it in farther.

Ensure top of padding is level with top of hook

3 Bandage over the padding and the hook; take care not to press down on the hook. See that the victim receives medical attention as soon as possible.

FOREIGN OBJECT IN THE EYE

A speck of dust, a loose eyelash, or even a contact lens can float on the white of the eye. Usually, such objects can easily be rinsed off. However, you must not touch anything that sticks to the eye, penetrates the eyeball, or rests on the colored part of the eye (iris and pupil) because this may damage the eye. Instead, make sure that the victim gets medical attention quickly.

 See also EYE WOUND p.65

✚ YOUR AIM
- To prevent injury to the eye.

❶ CAUTION

Do not touch anything that is sticking to, or embedded in, the eyeball or over the colored part of the eye. Cover the eye (see EYE WOUND, p.65) and take or send the victim to the hospital.

1 Advise the victim to sit down facing the light; tell her not to rub her eye. Stand behind the victim.

2 Gently separate her eyelids with your finger and thumb. Examine every part of her eye carefully.

Ask her to look right, left, up, and down

3 If you can see a foreign object on the white of the eye, wash it out by pouring clean water from a glass or by using a sterile eyewash.

Pour water on inner corner of eye

Let water drain on to towel

4 If this is unsuccessful, lift the object off with a moist swab or the damp corner of a tissue. If you still cannot remove the object, seek medical help.

SPECIAL CASE

OBJECT UNDER UPPER EYELID
Ask the victim to grasp her lashes and pull the upper lid over the lower lid. Blinking under water may also make the object float off.

Lower lashes may brush particle clear

FOREIGN OBJECT IN THE EAR

If a foreign object becomes lodged in the ear, it may block the ear canal and cause temporary deafness. In some cases, a foreign object may damage the eardrum. Young children frequently push objects into their ears. Insects can also fly or crawl into the ear and may cause alarm.

YOUR AIMS

- To prevent injury to the ear.
- To remove a trapped insect if it is moving.
- To arrange transportation to the hospital if a foreign object is lodged in the ear.

1 Arrange to take or send the victim to the hospital. Do not try to remove a lodged foreign object yourself.

2 Reassure the victim during the journey or until medical help arrives.

⚠ CAUTION

Do not attempt to remove any object that is lodged in the ear. You may cause serious injury and push the object in even farther.

SPECIAL CASE

INSECT INSIDE THE EAR
Reassure the victim, and ask her to sit down. Gently flood the ear with tepid water so that the insect floats out. If this flooding does not remove the insect, take or send the victim to the hospital.

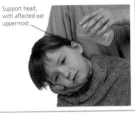

Support head, with affected ear uppermost

FOREIGN OBJECT IN THE NOSE

Young children may push small objects up their noses. Foreign objects can block the nose and cause infection. Sharp objects may damage the tissues, and "button" batteries can cause burns and bleeding. Do not try to remove a foreign object; you may cause injury.

RECOGNITION

There may be:
- Difficult/noisy breathing through the nose.
- Swelling of the nose.
- Smelly/blood-stained discharge, indicating that an object has been lodged for a while.

YOUR AIM

- To arrange transportation to the hospital.

⚠ CAUTION

Do not attempt to remove the foreign object, even if you can see it.

1 Keep the victim calm. Tell him to breathe through his mouth at a normal rate. Advise him not to poke inside his nose to try to remove the object himself.

2 Arrange to take or send the victim to the hospital, where the object can safely be removed by medical staff.

INHALED FOREIGN OBJECT

Small, smooth objects can slip past protective mechanisms in the throat and enter the air passages to the lungs. Dry peanuts, which can swell up when in contact with body fluids, pose a danger in young children; they can be inhaled into the lungs, resulting in serious damage.

People who are allergic to nuts may suffer anaphylactic shock (p.52) after swallowing them.

▶ Treat as for CHOKING ADULT p.46
• CHOKING CHILD p.47 • CHOKING
INFANT p.48

SWALLOWED FOREIGN OBJECT

Small objects such as coins, safety pins, or buttons are often swallowed by young children. They usually travel straight through the digestive tract, but there is a risk that they may enter the respiratory tract and cause choking.

Button batteries, used in some toys, watches, and hearing aids, contain corrosive chemicals; if swallowed, they can cause severe damage, and even death, if not removed. A large or sharp object may damage the digestive tract.

✚ YOUR AIM

- To obtain medical aid if necessary.

1 Reassure the victim and try to find out exactly what she has swallowed.

❶ WARNING

If the victim has swallowed something large or sharp, or has difficulty breathing or swallowing

DIAL 9·1·1 OR CALL EMS

Reassure the victim while waiting for medical help to arrive.

❶ CAUTION

Do not allow the victim to eat, drink, or smoke because a general anesthetic may need to be given in the hospital.

2 If the swallowed object is small and smooth, arrange to take or send the victim to the hospital or to see a doctor. Always seek urgent medical advice if you know or suspect that a victim has swallowed a battery.

9

POISONING IS USUALLY unintentional. It may result from exposure to or ingestion of toxic substances, including drugs and alcohol, chemicals, and contaminated food. Some cases of poisoning are intentional, as in cases of attempted suicide. The effects of a poison vary depending on the type and the amount of the substance absorbed. However, in most cases of poisoning, medical aid will be needed.

BITES AND STINGS
Insect stings are often minor injuries that can be treated with first aid. However, multiple insect stings can produce a very serious reaction that requires urgent medical help. Animal and human bites always need medical attention because the mouth harbors many microorganisms (germs).

CONTENTS

POISONING, BITES, AND STINGS

➕ FIRST-AID PRIORITIES

• Assess victim's condition.

• Identify the poisonous substance and call Poison Control Center (800-222-1222) for treatment information.

• Ensure safety of yourself and victim.

• Obtain medical aid if necessary. Dial 9·1·1 or call EMS if you suspect a serious illness or injury.

SWALLOWED POISONS

Chemicals that are swallowed may harm the digestive tract, or cause more widespread damage if they enter the bloodstream. Hazardous chemicals include common household substances such as bleach, dishwasher detergent, and paint thinner.

Drugs, whether prescribed or bought over the counter, are also potentially harmful if they are taken in overdose. The effects of poisoning depend on the substance that has been swallowed.

RECOGNITION

Depends on the poison, but there may be:

- Vomiting, sometimes bloodstained.
- Impaired consciousness.
- Pain or burning sensation.
- Empty containers in the vicinity.
- History of ingestion/exposure.

▶ See also CHEMICAL BURN p.103
● DRUG POISONING p.119 ● LIFE-SAVING PROCEDURES pp.19–48

YOUR AIMS

- To maintain the airway, breathing, and circulation.
- To remove any contaminated clothing.
- To identify the poison.
- To arrange urgent removal to the hospital.

SPECIAL CASE

BURNED LIPS
If the victim's lips are burned by corrosive substances, give her cold milk or water to rinse her mouth while waiting for medical help.

1 If the victim is conscious, ask her what she has swallowed, and try to reassure her.

Look for clues such as empty containers

⚠ WARNING

- Never attempt to induce vomiting.
- If the victim becomes unconscious, open the airway and check breathing; be prepared to give rescue breaths and chest compressions if necessary (*see* LIFE-SAVING PROCEDURES, pp.19–48). If she is breathing, place her in the recovery position (pp.30–31).

- Use a face shield or pocket mask (p.24) for rescue breathing if there are any chemicals on the victim's mouth.

2 CALL THE POISON CONTROL CENTER (800) 222-1222
Give as much information as possible about the swallowed poison, to help doctors to give appropriate treatment once the victim reaches the hospital.

DRUG POISONING

Poisoning can result from an overdose of either prescribed drugs or drugs that are bought over the counter. It can also be caused by drug abuse or drug interaction. The effects vary depending on the type of drug and how it is taken (below). When you call the Poison Control Center, give as much information as possible.

▶ See also LIFE-SAVING PROCEDURES pp.19–48

RECOGNITION

Category	Drug	Effects of poisoning
Analgesics	Aspirin (swallowed)	Upper abdominal pain, nausea, and vomiting ● Ringing in the ears ● "Sighing" when breathing ● Confusion and delirium ● Dizziness
	Acetaminophen (swallowed)	Little effect at first, but abdominal pain, nausea, and vomiting may develop ● Irreversible liver damage may occur within 3 days (malnourishment and alcohol increase the risk)
Nervous system depressants and tranquilizers	Barbiturates and benzodiazepines (swallowed)	Lethargy and sleepiness, leading to unconsciousness ● Shallow breathing ● Weak, irregular, or abnormally slow or fast pulse
Stimulants and hallucinogens	Amphetamines (including Ecstasy) and LSD (swallowed); cocaine (inhaled)	Excitable, hyperactive behavior, wildness, and frenzy ● Sweating ● Tremor of the hands ● Hallucinations, in which the victim may claim to "hear voices" or "see things"
Opioids	Morphine, heroin (commonly injected)	Small pupils ● Sluggishness and confusion, possibly leading to unconsciousness ● Slow, shallow breathing, which may stop altogether ● Needle marks, which may be infected
Solvents	Glue, lighter fuel (inhaled)	Nausea and vomiting ● Headaches ● Hallucinations ● Possibly, unconsciousness ● Rarely, cardiac arrest

➕ YOUR AIMS

● To maintain breathing and circulation.

● To arrange removal to the hospital.

ⓘ WARNING

● If the victim is unconscious, open the airway and check breathing; be prepared to give rescue breaths and chest compressions if necessary (see LIFE-SAVING PROCEDURES, pp.19–48). If breathing, place in the recovery position (pp.30–31).

DIAL 9·1·1 OR CALL EMS

● Do not induce vomiting.

1 If the victim is conscious, help him into a comfortable position and ask what he has taken. Reassure him while you talk to him.

2 CALL THE POISON CONTROL CENTER (800) 222-1222
Monitor and record vital signs – level of response, pulse, and breathing (pp.8–9) – until medical help arrives.

3 Keep samples of any vomited material. Look for evidence to help identify the drug, such as empty containers. Give samples and containers to the EMS crew.

ALCOHOL POISONING

Prolonged or excessive intake of alcohol (chemical name, ethanol) can severely impair all physical and mental functions, and the person may sink into deep unconsciousness.

There are several risks to the victim from alcohol poisoning:

- An unconscious victim risks inhaling and choking on vomit.
- Alcohol widens (dilates) the blood vessels. Consequently, the body loses heat, and hypothermia may develop.
- A victim who smells of alcohol may be misdiagnosed and not be treated appropriately for an underlying cause of unconsciousness, such as a head injury, stroke, or heart attack.

RECOGNITION

There may be:
- A strong smell of alcohol.
- Impaired consciousness: the victim may respond if roused, but will quickly relapse.
- Flushed and moist face.
- Deep, noisy breathing.
- Full, bounding pulse.
- Unconsciousness.

In the later stages of unconsciousness:
- Dry, bloated appearance to the face.
- Shallow breathing.
- Weak, rapid pulse.
- Dilated pupils that react poorly to light.

See also HYPOTHERMIA pp.108–110
LIFE-SAVING PROCEDURES pp.19–48

YOUR AIMS

- To maintain an open airway.
- To assess for other conditions.
- To seek medical help if necessary.

WARNING

- If the victim is unconscious, open the airway and check breathing; be prepared to give rescue breaths and start chest compressions if necessary (see LIFE-SAVING PROCEDURES, pp.19–48). If the victim is breathing, place him in the recovery position (pp.30–31).

DIAL 9·1·1 OR CALL EMS

- Do not induce vomiting.

1 Cover the victim with a coat or blanket to protect him from the cold.

2 Assess the victim for any injuries, especially head injuries, or other medical conditions.

3 Regularly monitor and record vital signs – level of response, pulse, and breathing (pp.8–9) – until the victim recovers or can be placed in the care of a responsible person.

Watch victim in case he becomes unconscious

Put a coat or blanket over him

FOOD POISONING

This is usually caused by consuming food or drink that is contaminated with bacteria or viruses. Some food poisoning is caused by poisons (toxins) from bacteria already in the food. Symptoms may develop within hours, or they may not occur until a day or so after eating contaminated food.

Toxic food poisoning is frequently caused by poisons produced by the staphylococcus group of bacteria. Symptoms usually develop rapidly, possibly within 2–6 hours of eating the affected food.

One danger of food poisoning is loss of body fluids. The dehydration

RECOGNITION

There may be:
- Nausea and vomiting.
- Cramping abdominal pains.
- Diarrhea (possibly blood-stained).
- Headache or fever.
- Features of shock (p.50).
- Impaired consciousness.

that results can be serious if fluids are not replaced quickly. Dehydration is especially serious in the very young and the very old, and, in some cases, hospital treatment may be required.

▶ See also SHOCK pp.50–51

YOUR AIMS
- To encourage the victim to rest.
- To give the victim plenty of bland fluids to drink.
- To obtain medical aid if necessary.

WARNING
If the victim's condition worsens, **DIAL 9·1·1 OR CALL EMS**

1 Advise the victim to lie down and rest. Help her if necessary.

2 Give the victim small amounts of bland fluids to drink and a bowl to use if she vomits. Call a doctor for advice.

3 Slowly give more fluids after vomiting stops.

Give bland fluids such as water, diluted fruit juice, or weak tea

Cover victim to keep her comfortable

Give victim a bowl to use if she feels nauseous

INSECT STING

Usually, a sting from a bee, wasp, or hornet is painful but not dangerous. However, multiple insect stings or a sting in the mouth or throat can produce a serious reaction. With any bite or sting, watch for signs of an allergic reaction, which may lead to anaphylactic shock (p.52).

RECOGNITION

• Pain at the site of the sting.

• Redness and swelling around the site of the sting.

▶ See also ANAPHYLACTIC SHOCK p.52

• LIFE-SAVING PROCEDURES pp.19–48

YOUR AIMS

• To relieve swelling and pain.

• To arrange removal to hospital if needed.

⚠ WARNING

If the victim shows signs of anaphylactic shock, such as impaired breathing or swelling of the face and neck,

DIAL 9·1·1 OR CALL EMS

1 If the sting is visible, brush or scrape it off sideways with your fingernail, a credit card, or the blunt edge of a knife. Do not use tweezers; more poison may be injected into the victim.

Brush sting off with a fingernail or blunt edge

2 Raise the affected part if possible, and apply an ice pack or cold compress (p.12) for at least 10 minutes. Advise the victim to see her doctor if the pain and swelling persist.

SPECIAL CASE

STINGS TO THE MOUTH AND THROAT

If a victim has been stung in the mouth, the mouth and/or throat may swell, causing blockage of the airway. To help prevent this, give the victim an ice cube to suck or cold water to sip. If swelling develops,

DIAL 9·1·1 OR CALL EMS

Cold water helps to reduce risk of swelling

TICK BITE

Ticks are tiny, spiderlike creatures that attach themselves to passing animals (including humans) and bite into the skin to suck blood. Ticks can carry disease and cause infection, so they should be removed as soon as possible.

YOUR AIM

• To remove the tick.

1 Using fine-pointed tweezers, grasp the tick's head close to the victim's skin.

2 Use a to-and-fro action to lever the head out. Try to avoid breaking the tick and leaving the buried head behind.

3 Advise the victim to see a doctor as soon as possible.

SNAKE BITE

The only poisonous snakes native to the US are pit vipers (such as rattlesnakes) and coral snakes. More exotic poisonous snakes may be kept as pets. A snake bite is often not serious, but can be frightening. The victim should keep still to delay the spread of venom through the body. Note the snake's appearance to help doctors give the correct antivenom. Bear in mind that venom is active even if the snake is dead. If it safe to do so, put the snake in a secure container.

Depends on the species, but there may be;
- A pair of puncture marks.
- Severe pain, redness, and swelling at the site of the bite.
- Nausea, vomiting, disturbed vision.
- Increased salivation and sweating.
- Labored breathing; in extreme cases, breathing may stop altogether.

See also LIFE-SAVING PROCEDURES pp.19–48

YOUR AIMS
- To prevent the spread of venom.
- To arrange urgent removal to the hospital.

WARNING
- Do not apply a tourniquet, slash the wound with a knife, or suck out the venom.
- If the victim becomes unconscious, open the airway and check breathing; be prepared to give rescue breaths and chest compressions if necessary (see LIFE-SAVING PROCEDURES, pp.19–48).

1 Help the victim lie down. Reassure her, and tell her to keep calm and still. DIAL 9·1·1 OR CALL EMS

2 Gently wash the wound and pat dry with clean swabs.

Clean wound with gauze swab

3 Lightly compress the limb above the wound with a roller bandage. Use triangular bandages to immobilize the affected area (p.16).

Tie cravat bandage in figure-eight around feet

Keep heart above the level of wounded part

Leave bite exposed

Binder bandage | Soft padding | Roller bandage

ANIMAL BITE

Bites from sharp, pointed teeth cause deep puncture wounds that can carry bacteria and other germs far into the tissues. Any bite that breaks the skin needs prompt medical attention because of the risk of infection.

The most serious infection risk is rabies, a potentially fatal virus that is carried in the saliva of infected animals. If bitten, the victim must receive antirabies injections. Tetanus is also a potential risk following any animal bite. There is probably only a small risk of hepatitis B or C viruses being transmitted through a human bite – and an even smaller risk of transmission of the HIV (AIDS) virus. However, seek medical advice if you are concerned.

⊙ See also CUTS AND SCRAPES p.62
● SEVERE BLEEDING pp.60–61 ● SHOCK pp.50–51

✚ YOUR AIMS

- To control bleeding.
- To minimize the risk of infection, both to the victim and yourself.
- To obtain medical aid if necessary.

❶ CAUTION

Always ask about tetanus immunization.
Seek medical advice if:
- The victim has never been immunized.
- The victim is uncertain about the timing or number of injections that have been given.
- It is more than 10 years since the victim's last injection.

1 Put on disposable gloves if available. Wash the bite wound thoroughly with soap and warm water in order to minimize the risk of infection.

2 Pat dry with clean gauze swabs and cover with an adhesive bandage or a small sterile dressing.

Dry around wound

3 Take or send the victim to the hospital if the wound is large or deep.

❶ WARNING

If you suspect rabies, take or send the victim to the hospital immediately.

SPECIAL CASE

DEEP WOUND
If the wound is deep, control bleeding by applying direct pressure and raising the injured part. Cover the wound with a nonfluffy pad, or a sterile wound dressing, and bandage in place to control bleeding. Take or send the victim to the hospital.

Cover wound and bandage firmly

Raise injured part

INDEX

AMERICAN COLLEGE OF EMERGENCY PHYSICIANS

Americans make almost 100 million visits to hospital emergency departments each year seeking treatment for everything from heart attacks and strokes to cuts and sprains. The American College of Emergency Physicians (ACEP) has been representing the doctors who provide that care for more than 30 years. Our goal from the beginning has been to support high-quality emergency care – especially by providing education and information. The American College of Emergency Physicians *Pocket First Aid* should be in every household, car, and backpack. This manual shows you what you can do, by yourself, to properly deal with many common injuries, and how to assist seriously injured or ill individuals while you wait for medical assistance. It explains treatments and techniques in a step-by-step manner and demonstrates with hundreds of photographs exactly how to perform them correctly.

Using the proper first-aid techniques can be crucial in an emergency situation. As emergency physicians who treat thousands of patients a year, we have seen many situations where providing the right care at the right time has made all the difference.

ACEP was founded by physicians who realized that, in order to provide emergency care, a doctor must master a unique body of knowledge and emergency skills. Specialists in emergency medicine play an ever-increasing role in meeting the emergency health care needs of our country. With the leadership provided by ACEP and the 22,000 emergency physicians the College represents, America has the best and most advanced emergency medical care in the world.

On behalf of the American College of Emergency Physicians and the dedicated emergency medicine specialists who provide care in hospital emergency departments throughout the country, we are very proud to introduce *Pocket First Aid* to you.

Michael T. Rapp, MD FACEP
President, American College of Emergency
Physicians, 1999–2000

Jon R. Krohmer, MD FACEP, Medical Editor

Tom Werlinich, Associate Executive Director
of Educational and Professional Publications

OBSERVATION CHARTS

Fill in the charts below when you attend a victim. On the first chart, place a dot opposite the appropriate score at each time interval. On the second, check the appropriate pulse and breathing rates at each interval.

LEVEL OF RESPONSE CHART

DATE............................ VICTIM'S NAME............................

OBSERVATION	RESPONSE/SCORE	Time of observation (minutes)					
		0	10	20	30	40	50
Eyes Observe for reaction while testing other responses.	Open spontaneously **4** Open to speech **3** Open to painful stimulus **2** No response **1**						
Speech When testing responses, speak clearly and directly, close to victim's ear.	Responds sensibly to questions **5** Seems confused **4** Uses inappropriate words **3** Incomprehensible sounds **2** No response **1**						
Movement Apply painful stimulus: pinch ear lobe or skin on back of hand.	Obeys commands **6** Points to pain **5** Withdraws from painful stimulus **4** Bends limbs in response to pain **3** Straightens limbs in response to pain **2** No response **1**						
	TOTAL SCORE						

PULSE AND BREATHING CHECK CHART

DATE............................ VICTIM'S NAME............................

PULSE/BREATHING	RATE	Time of observation (minutes)					
		0	10	20	30	40	50
Pulse (beats per minute) Take pulse at wrist or at neck on adult, or at inner arm on baby (p.8). Note the rate, and whether beats are weak (w) or strong (s), regular (reg) or irregular (irreg).	Over 110						
	101–110						
	91–100						
	81–90						
	71–80						
	61–70						
	Below 61						
Breathing (breaths per minute) Note rate, and whether breathing is quiet (q) or noisy (n), easy (e) or difficult (diff).	Over 40						
	31–40						
	21–30						
	11–20						
	Below 20						
	TOTAL SCORE						